D1602429

A CRITIQUE OF
NICOTINE ADDICTION

A CRITIQUE OF
NICOTINE ADDICTION

by

Hanan Frenk
The Academic College of Tel Aviv-Yafo
&
Tel-Aviv University

and

Reuven Dar
Tel Aviv University

KLUWER ACADEMIC PUBLISHERS
Boston / Dordrecht / London

Distributors for North, Central and South America:
Kluwer Academic Publishers
101 Philip Drive
Assinippi Park
Norwell, Massachusetts 02061 USA
Telephone (781) 871-6600
Fax (781) 681-9045
E-Mail <kluwer@wkap.com>

Distributors for all other countries:
Kluwer Academic Publishers Group
Distribution Centre
Post Office Box 322
3300 AH Dordrecht, THE NETHERLANDS
Telephone 31 78 6392 392
Fax 31 78 6546 474
E-Mail <services@wkap.nl>

 Electronic Services <http://www.wkap.nl>

Library of Congress Cataloging-in-Publication Data

Frenk, Hanan.
    A critique of nicotine addiction / by Hanan Frenk and Reuvan Dar.
      p.cm.—(Neurobiological foundation of aberrant behaviors; 2)
      Includes bibliographical references and index.
      ISBN 0-7923-7225-5 (alk. paper)
        1. Tobacco habit. 2. Smoking—Health aspects. I. Dar, Reuven, 1954- II. Title. III
    Neurobiological foundation of aberrant behaviors; 2

    RC567 .F728 2000
    616.86'5—dc21   00-062206

Printed on acid-free paper.

Printed in the United States of America

The Publisher offers discounts on this book for course use and bulk purchases. For further information, send email to <michael.williams@wkap.com>.

Contents

Foreword

In her book, *'Defenders of the Truth'*, Ullica Segerstrale posed a rhetorical question, What makes a hardcover academic book a hot seller: "How does one convince academics and the general public that this is a book that they absolutely need to have?". The prospects are surely increased by an intriguing name, an appealing cover, when a book is loaded with full-page drawings, and if its price is satisfactory. However, in the recipe for success these are all necessary, but not sufficient ingredients: "The answer", she submits, "is, of course, controversy". If we trust her judgment, the book by H. Frenk and R. Dar is the right book to succeed. It is about nicotine, the topic where the battle lines are long drawn. The authors marshaled convincing evidence that nicotine is not addictive, and that proponents of nicotine addiction barked up the wrong tree. It rubs many influential opponents the wrong way, and it is published in a climate after the Florida nicotine trial. Recommending this scholarly book to a reader I have to caution him not to misunderstand its message. It is not against potential dangers of smoking, nor does it argue that nicotine is a worthy substance to use, even if some of its effects are salubrious and can be employed in medicine. It is only about the addictive potential of nicotine or rather, it is about the fact that the passion with which debates are conducted in science may vary inversely with the depth of knowledge on which convictions are based.

Michael Myslobodsky

Acknowledgements

We would like to thank Zalman Amit and Robert E. Lubow for their insightful comments on various parts of this manuscript. This in no way implies that these friends and colleagues agree with any of the opinions expressed in this book. We are also grateful for the invaluable assistance of Yafa Shaar, Chaya Amir and Liel Rubinsky in preparing the manuscript. Most of all, we are eternally indebted to our life companions, Levanna and Rachelli, for tolerating our tiresome single-mindedness for such a long time.

H.F. wishes to dedicate this book to the memory of John Liebeskind, a friend and mentor, who left a void that remains unfilled.

R.D. wishes to dedicate this book to the memory of his mother, Ruthie, the first person he would have liked to share it with.

Chapter 1

INTRODUCTION

Is nicotine an addictive drug? The mere raising of this question today would seem preposterous to both scientists and lay people, smokers and non-smokers alike. When we embarked on writing this book, friends and colleagues responded with astonishment and dismay. They did not want to see us ruin our modest reputation, and referred us kindly to recent scientific reviews[635], and to public statements by the Surgeon General[665] and the British Royal College of Physicians[42,43,534,657,657]. These respected authorities not only agreed that nicotine was the addictive drug that caused smoking, but declared that it was at least as addictive as heroine and cocaine. One of the (anonymous) expert referees of this book began his review thus: "*The proposed book ...really caught my attention by the almost unheard of premise that nicotine is not addictive. My initial impression of this view was that Drs. Frenk and Dar may have been smoking some substances other than tobacco.*" Clearly, to our colleagues as well as to the majority of the scientific community, nicotine addiction is no longer a theory which can be legitimately questioned.

1.   NICOTINE ADDICTION: FACT OR THEORY?

Facts, in non-positivistic science, are theories that have acquired a status of unchallenged empirical statements[363]. Nicotine addiction, according to this criterion, has become a fact. In the vast majority of research articles and reviews concerning smoking, it is indeed stated as a matter of fact rather than a hypothesis with evidence for and against it. Countless research papers begin with variations of the sentences "*Nicotine is the active ingredient in tobacco that leads to addiction*[621] (p. 221)" or "*The reinforcement provided by nicotine is a necessary component of the processes that drive smoking behavior*[148] (p. 83)," providing, as a sole reference, the 1988 Report of the Surgeon General.

The "*near-consensus*" that nicotine is addictive, as Stolerman and Jarvis[635] put it, "*was enshrined in the 1988 report of the Surgeon General, which regarded nicotine addictive in the same sense as drugs such as heroin and cocaine* (p.117)." This "enshrined" status seems to have relieved investigators from the scientific obligation of skepticism, and not only in the USA. A recent report on nicotine addiction in Britain[657], which purports to provide an updated and objective review of the evidence for nicotine addiction, provides instead an uncritical endorsement of the view "enshrined" by the Surgeon General. Its "*central conclusion*" repeats the Surgeon General's[665] statement almost word to word (p. 183): "*The central conclusion of this report is that cigarette smoking should be understood as a manifestation of nicotine addiction, and that the extent to which smokers are addicted to nicotine is comparable with addiction to 'hard' drugs such as heroin and cocaine.*" Notice the decisive tone of the paragraph that follows this 'conclusion:' "*Nicotine is an addictive drug, and the primary purpose of smoking tobacco is to deliver a dose of nicotine rapidly to receptors in the brain. This generates a pleasurable sensation for the smoker which, with repeated experience, rapidly consolidates into physiological and psychological addiction reinforced by pronounced withdrawal symptoms.*"

As we hope to show in this book, the unwavering assuredness in which statements about nicotine addiction are typically made is entirely unjustified by available data. We submit that an objective evaluation of these data leads to the conclusion that nicotine is not an addictive drug and that the popularized equation of the addictive properties of nicotine and heroin has little to do with science.

2.   WHAT THIS BOOK IS NOT ABOUT

Smoking has been blamed for the death of millions and for compromising the quality of life of many more. It has been the subject of dramatic legal battles, social and political debate, media interest and personal and family conflicts. It is therefore not surprising that it is almost impossible to discuss smoking dispassionately. Nevertheless, as we began to discuss the arguments presented in this book, we were surprised at the emotional responses that our claims generated even in the most professional audiences. We repeatedly found, once these highly charged responses were clarified, that our claims have been entirely misunderstood. This pattern has indicated to us that it would be essential to elucidate what it is exactly we are claiming in this book, and more importantly, what it is exactly that we are *not* claiming.

The most important point to stress is that there is nothing in what we are about to argue that should be interpreted as supporting the habit of smoking or discounting the difficulty of quitting. By claiming that nicotine is not an addictive drug we are not saying that smoking is easy to quit, and certainly not that it is a healthy habit. These points are crucial for a correct interpretation of our position. We shall start with the second point, which may be the easier one to clarify; but first, we should define briefly some basic terms that we shall use throughout the book.

Cigarette smoke consists of a volatile phase, which includes a large variety of gaseous compounds, and a particulate phase, which includes an even larger number of compounds. The particulate matter, without its alkaloid and water content, is referred to as "tar[657]." Nicotine is the major compound in the particulate phase of cigarette smoke. During smoking, small droplets of tar, which also contain nicotine, are deposited in the small airways and the nicotine is absorbed into the bloodstream and distributed throughout the body[657].

There are many compounds in cigarette smoke that have been identified as health risks. These include gaseous compounds such as CO, nitrogen and ammonia, and known carcinogens such as polynuclear aromatic hydrocarbons, N-nitrosamines and aromatic amines which are found in the "tar." There is consensus among researchers that the health-risks associated with smoking, including cancer, respiratory illnesses, circulatory diseases etc., are associated with these compounds, rather than with nicotine.

Nothing in the ideas we develop in this book suggests that smoking is healthier than what is commonly believed. On this issue we are not making any judgment simply because we are not qualified to do so. We lack the necessary medical training and we are certainly not adequately familiar with the relevant research. On a personal level, we accept the prevailing view that smoking is associated with serious health risks. We believe it would be rational for everyone to avoid or minimize smoking because of the its short- and long-term effects on health. The issue of whether or not nicotine is addictive has nothing to do with this belief, however. As noted above, even those who argue that nicotine is the drug in cigarettes that causes addiction blame nicotine not for direct ill-effects on health but for its presumed role in maintaining smoking[e.g.,657].

While it may be acceptable to most readers that the question of nicotine addiction has nothing to do with the health risks associated with smoking, the second point we are stressing may be more difficult to swallow. It seems self-evident that in questioning the notion that nicotine is an addictive drug, we are in effect suggesting that smoking is easy to quit. We want to dispute this interpretation as emphatically as we can. As we shall show throughout this book, many habits that do not involve psychoactive drugs are extremely difficult to break. These include pathological gambling, compulsive stealing (kleptomania), binge eating and other habits that may be at least as damaging as smoking. Thus, as we show later, the conclusion that the difficulty of quitting smoking testifies for the validity of the nicotine addiction hypothesis is as false as it is seductive.

Returning to the personal level, we differ from each other in our attitudes toward smoking and our personal experience with it. The first author is presently a light smoker and a past heavy smoker as well as a serial ex-smoker. The second author never smoked and is passionately averse to being around people who do, the first author included. We note this to emphasize that in arguing that nicotine is not addictive, we have no intention of praising the merits of smoking.

3.   WHAT THIS BOOK *IS* ABOUT, AND WHO CARES?

Having clarified what we are not saying in this book, let us state what we *are* saying. This book is a critique of the nicotine addiction hypothesis, based on a critical examination of the research literature commonly believed to prove that nicotine is addicting. Put simply, we claim that on present evidence, there is every reason to reject the generally accepted theory that nicotine causes smoking, or that the difficulty in quitting is caused by nicotine.

Several colleagues, who heard about our plan to publish this book, had this reaction: *"Who cares whether nicotine plays a role in smoking or not? Everyone knows that it is difficult to stop smoking, so what difference does it make if nicotine is the cause of this difficulty? The important thing is that people quit smoking, and your book won't help."* This perspective is quite common. In fact, one of the explicit goals of declaring that smoking was a chemical addiction was the perception that this would help the fight against smoking[e.g.,657]. We beg to differ with this view. We believe that the need to fight smoking is one of the most important reasons to question the nicotine addiction hypothesis. Several studies demonstrated that the more smokers believe that they are addicted, the more difficult they perceive quitting to be[321,334,407] and the less confident they are about their own chances of quitting[160,161]. Moreover, the belief that smoking is an addiction seems to be a self-fulfilling prophecy, as it is associated with shorter duration of cessation attempts and higher relapse rates[470]. It seems that smokers' belief that they are addicted leads to an external attribution of control over smoking and undermines their sense of self-efficacy[30]. If the present book contributes to a different perception of smoking, namely that smoking is a controllable habit and nicotine is not an addictive drug, it may well enhance not only smokers' belief in their ability to quit but their actual ability to do so.

Furthermore, practically all present plans regarding the fight against smoking and the regulation of tobacco products is based on the assumption that cigarettes are basically nicotine delivery devices[265,657]. If nicotine is in fact not an addictive drug and is has little to do with why people smoke cigarettes, this would have major implication for public policies designed to counter the risks associated with smoking. For example, a recent report of the British Royal College of Physicians[657] makes the following recommendation: *"The phenomenon of nicotine dependence is heavily entrenched in society. It is obviously desirable to reduce both nicotine dependence and the terrible harm caused by nicotine delivery through tobacco smoke, but it may be necessary to accept, albeit reluctantly, the intractability of widespread nicotine dependence in the short to medium term. In this case, product development that enable nicotine users to take nicotine with less harm to their health should be encouraged...* (p. 187)." Of course, such a recommendation makes no sense if nicotine is not the reason that people smoke cigarettes. Finally, a major motivation for writing this book is to counter some of the negative effects that the broad consensus regarding nicotine addiction has had on relevant research.

As we show throughout our review of the literature, the research on nicotine addiction has been replete with severe methodological errors, including systematic exclusion of uncooperative subjects, use of preconditioned subjects, and a staggering under-utilization of crucial control conditions. We are convinced that these problems reflect a prevailing bias in this area, rather than researchers' inaptitude. The decision to use control groups, for example, is inversely related to the plausibility of the hypothesis under study. The near-consensus "enshrined" in the 1988 Report of the Surgeon General has boosted the subjective plausibility of nicotine addiction to such extent that the need for excluding alternative explanations by the use of appropriate control groups has diminished. In the same vein, counter-evidence has been systematically discounted or even ignored by the scientific community and even more so by government officials such as the Surgeon General. Alternative explanation of existing data have rarely been raised, even when these alternative explanations were not only viable but immanently plausible and parsimonious.

In the opening lines of his article, "The dark side of religion," M.R. Cohen (p. 279) wrote: *"The advocatus diaboli, as you know, is not a lawyer employed by the Prince of Darkness. He is a faithful member of the Church whose duty it is, when it is proposed to canonize a saint, to search out all the opposing considerations and to state them as cogently as possible. This wise institution compels the advocates of canonization to exert themselves to develop arguments vigorous enough to overcome all objections[107]."* Together with modern philosophers of science[365,502], we believe that the growth of science and our faith in the scientific method depend on an attitude of continued criticism. When this critical attitude is relaxed, science may turn into propaganda. The purpose of this book is to reverse this trend and return a healthy measure of doubt to the nicotine addiction hypothesis.

4.   AN OUTLINE OF THE BOOK

Next, in Chapter 2, we discuss three related terms: addiction, compulsion and habit. We begin with the classic pharmacological definition of addiction and move on to the modern behavioral definition as exemplified by the diagnostic criteria of the American Psychiatric Association[10]and the World Health Organization[711]. We proceed to explore the similarity between the current definition of addiction and the phenomenology of habits, particularly compulsive habits. We show that habits share with addictions the features of persistence, craving, 'withdrawal symptoms' upon cessation and a high rate of relapse. Therefore, these criteria are insufficient to define drug addictions (or 'substance dependence') from compulsions that do not involve psychoactive substances.

In Chapter 3 we distinguish various ways in which psychoactive substances may be used habitually. We begin by demonstrating that the habitual use of psychoactive drugs (including caffeine, alcohol, and nicotine) is almost universal in our society. Nevertheless, only a minority of users can be reasonably claimed to be addicted to these substances. We show that habits that involve psychoactive drugs can be divided into several types, distinguished by the role the drug plays in motivating or maintaining the habit. The chapter concludes with our 'drug attribution bias' hypothesis, which postulates that when a habit involves consumption of a psychoactive substance, observers will tend to attribute the habit to the substance even when, in reality, it may have absolutely no role in maintaining the habit.

Chapter 4 begins with the Surgeon General's 1988 declaration that smoking is a form of drug addiction and that "*nicotine is the drug in tobacco that causes addiction*[665]." We review the Surgeon General's definition of drug dependence and its implications for testing the nicotine addiction hypothesis. We show that most of his criteria for drug dependence are nonspecific, in that they do not distinguish drug-driven from other compulsive habits. According to the Surgeon General's definition, neither physical dependence nor tolerance are necessary criteria for drug dependence, and the only required causal relationship between the drug and the behavior is the requirement that the drug should be capable of directly reinforcing behavior. Therefore, testing the nicotine addiction hypothesis essentially reduces to testing whether nicotine is reinforcing.

We begin our exploration of the reinforcing effects of nicotine in Chapter 5, where we examine the theoretical and methodological foundations of the principal experimental paradigm in this area, namely the drug self-administration paradigm. We focus on factors that may confound interpretation of the results of animal self-administration studies, including the acquisition of secondary reinforcing properties by classic conditioning. In addition, we show that in studies of nicotine self-administration, careful control must be used to rule out alternative factors other than the reinforcing effects of nicotine, especially its non-specific activating effect.

In Chapter 6, we review the evidence for the proposition that nicotine is reinforcing for animals, including oral and intravenous self-administration studies and classical conditioning paradigms. We begin with the early nicotine self-administration studies, on which the Surgeon General based his claim that "*nicotine itself could function as an efficacious positive reinforcer for animals*[665]." A detailed analysis of these studies shows that they were fundamentally flawed and could not provide an empirical basis for the Surgeon General's claim. Proceeding to newer research, we illuminate blatant methodological errors, including lack of adequate controls and elimination of 'uncooperative' animals, which invalidate the results of the vast majority of these studies.

Chapter 7 examines another paradigm that purportedly provides empirical evidence for the nicotine addiction hypothesis, namely nicotine's effects on intracranial self-stimulation (ICSS). We show that on both theoretical and empirical grounds, ICSS has little value for determining the reinforcing properties of drugs, including nicotine. We also discuss briefly the dopamine hypothesis, as dopamine release is often cited as evidence for the claim that nicotine is rewarding. We summarize evidence that falsifies this hypothesis and specifically the equation of dopamine release with reward.

In Chapter 8, we step into the question that is more directly relevant to smoking, that is, whether nicotine is reinforcing to humans. We begin in a detailed critique of human self-administration studies and continue with a review of other nicotine administration studies in smokers and non-smokers.

We show that people do not enjoy nicotine injections, gums, patches, or intranasal spray and many suffer from symptoms such as nausea and vomiting, headaches and sleep disturbances. Nearly all nicotine administration studies, regardless of the route or speed of delivery, indicate that naive participants dislike nicotine. Whereas nicotine is generally less aversive to smokers or ex-smokers, this can be attributed to factors such as tolerance and acquired expectations, rather than the presumed reinforcing properties of nicotine. Finally, we review evidence in support of the possibility that smoking is motivated not by the psychactive effects of nicotine but by the pleasurable taste, smell, sensory and oral stimulation that smoking provides.

Chapter 9 focuses on the classic criteria of drug addiction, namely tolerance and physical dependence, and reviews the research pertaining to the notion that animals and humans develop tolerance to and physical dependence on nicotine. We show that in contrast to the cases of heroin and alcohol, neither humans nor animals show evidence of tolerance to the euphoric effects of nicotine. We proceed to review both animal and human research on physical dependence, and conclude that the observations concerning nicotine dependence in rats not only are highly problematic, but are also irrelevant to humans. We survey evidence that the smoking abstinence syndrome in humans can be abolished by cigarettes that do not contain nicotine, whereas pure nicotine reduces it only partially. Finally, we discuss research on ulcerative colitis, which shows that ex-smokers do not demonstrate any signs of dependence on nicotine even after prolonged exposure to nicotine at amounts comparable to the intake of an average smoker.

Chapter 10 explores the empirical basis for the Surgeon General's assertion that smoking abstinence rates are similar to those found for heroin and alcohol. We begin by showing that smokers have been remarkably compliant with smoking regulations, whereas outlawing heroin has totally failed to affect heroin use. We then demonstrate that the Surgeon General based his abstinence rate comparison only on short-term prospective studies, and that once retrospective data are considered, smoking cessation appears much more feasible and commonplace than cessation of heroin. Next, we argue that even if relapse rates of smoking were similar to those of heroin, the deduction that nicotine is as addictive as heroin does not follow, either logically or empirically. We compare the success and relapse rates reported in smoking cessation and in dieting, to show that the difficulty in abstaining from unhealthy habits does not depend on the presence of psychoactive drugs. Finally, we explore the role of motivation, a factor that is often disregarded or downplayed in smoking cessation research.

Chapter 11 is a discussion of the so-called "nicotine replacement" treatments, which are often cited as evidence for the nicotine addiction hypothesis. In this short chapter, we underscore two essential observations with regard to the "nicotine replacement treatment". Firstly, we show that the efficacy of such treatments is very modest, compared to many other non-chemical methods of smoking cessation. Secondly, a comparison with methadone maintenance treatment for heroin addiction shows that the presumed similarity between the two types of treatment is untenable, and that the two types of interventions evidently operate by entirely different mechanisms.

In chapter 12, we explore the tale of "nicotine compensation" or "nicotine titration," which holds that smokers titrate their smoking to obtain desired levels of nicotine. We review both switching studies and cross-sectional studies, which are typically cited as evidence for compensation. Based on these studies and related evidence, we argue that "nicotine titration" is a misnomer, and that whereas nicotine seems to be involved in down-regulation of smoking, it does not seem to have a role in up-regulation. Instead, up-regulation of smoking appears to be motivated by other aspects of the smoking habit, primarily by the sensory rewards of smoking. Paradoxically, our analysis of the evidence suggests that the only role nicotine has in determining smoking may be in imposing a ceiling on the extent or intensity of smoking. This effect is due not to the purported addictive properties of nicotine, but rather to its toxic effects.

Chapter 13 concludes the book. Its first sections are dedicated to a summary of our main contentions, including a table that compares the addictive properties of nicotine and heroin. The rest of the chapter is dedicated to an exploration of the scientific, social and political aspects of the nicotine addiction hypothesis. We demonstrate that the research on nicotine addiction has been characterized by a disturbing confirmatory bias and a degeneration of the scientific ideals of objectivity and skepticism. We relate these problems to several factors, primarily the "enshrined" status of the nicotine addiction hypothesis, which has deterred researchers, for a variety of reasons, from exploring dissenting views.

As stated earlier, we are fully aware of the broad consensus amongst professionals and laymen alike that nicotine is addictive, but the validity of scientific propositions is not established by popular vote but by evidence. We wrote this book to offer an opportunity to colleagues and laymen alike to evaluate the evidence from a different perspective than the one provided by consensual summaries. We invite the reader to relax his or her prejudices and review the original research, just as we did, with a skeptical eye.

Chapter 2

ADDICTION, COMPULSION, AND HABIT

Although many psychoactive drugs have been used by humans for hundreds and even thousands of years (for a historical review, see Brecher[62]), the term **drug addiction** was a creation of the twentieth century. Originally the word 'addiction' (from the Latin source, *addicere*) was used for a strong inclination towards any kind of conduct, good or bad[681]. Only towards the end of the nineteenth century did 'addiction' begin to be used to describe a preoccupation with drugs, but it still did not have the connotations that the term would receive later. Thus, when the German physician Levinstein wrote the first detailed description of opium addiction in 1877, he still saw addiction as a human passion, such as smoking, gambling, greediness for profit, sexual excesses, etc[51]. This may be related to the fact that opium and its derivatives, the opiates (e.g., heroin, morphine, and codeine), were openly and legally used in the USA until the beginning of the twentieth century and were considered by many less offensive than cigarette smoking[104]. The observation that opium caused less health damage than alcohol even led physicians in the USA to prescribe opium and morphine for alcoholics as a substitute for alcohol[62]. Thus, until the end of the 19th century, "*most physicians regarded addiction as a morbid appetite, a habit, or a vice[305].*" In fact, caffeine drew nearly as much concern as the opiates during that period[619].

The twentieth century gave the word 'addiction' a new meaning, that of an uncontrollable disease[384]. The word did not relate originally to opiates, but rather to alcohol. Alcoholism was perceived as a progressive disease, the chief symptom of which was a loss of control over drinking behavior and whose only remedy was abstinence from all alcoholic beverages[384]. The first of the psychoactive drugs, after alcohol, to be labeled "addictive" were the opiates, and they were subsequently outlawed in the USA by the Harrison Act in 1914. Alcohol was outlawed a few years later during the Prohibition, which lasted from 1920 to 1933. Since then, the label "addictive" has been attached to many other drugs. Barbiturates, benzodiazepines, cannabis, cocaine, LSD and many others – including of course tobacco and nicotine – all have been called "addictive" at one time or another, and the non-sanctioned use of most of them is forbidden nearly everywhere.

1.   PHARMACOLOGICAL DEFINITIONS OF ADDICTION

The view that addiction is a progressive disease proved to be scientifically useful when applied to some of the psychoactive drugs. Since the twenties, pharmacologists began to use the term for what is currently called **physical dependence**, namely the acquired physical need for drugs. They explained this need by drug-specific, progressive changes in the central nervous system which, ultimately, lead to an altered state where *not* taking the drug is highly unpleasant. This withdrawal, or abstinence, syndrome, which characterizes long-term use of drugs such as opiates, barbiturates, and alcohol, was assumed to be a primary motivation for continued drug use.

This, then, is what drug addiction meant to a prominent pharmacologist in the seventies[606]: "*...the most striking feature of narcotic addiction* [is] *the development of an apparent physiological requirement for a toxic foreign substance. As a result of this dependence the addicted animal seems to be "well" while intoxicated but becomes ill when the poison is removed. This illness is called the withdrawal syndrome* (p. 408)." As the cessation of many psychoactive drugs after long-term consumption is not followed by withdrawal symptoms, those drugs were not labeled "addictive." To distinguish the addictive from the non-addictive psychoactive drugs, a different term was coined to describe the latter category: "habitual drugs[710]." The concepts of addiction or physical dependence were therefore strictly defined within a biological context. They were not intended or used to describe *behaviors*: 'addictive' and 'habitual' were properties of *drugs*, and used accordingly as in 'addictive drugs' and 'habitual drugs.'

The unambiguous pharmacological definition of addiction, which hinged on the presence of drug-specific withdrawal symptoms, namely, on physical dependence, did not survive for long. Over the past 30 years, there has been a clear trend of expansion of the term 'addiction' or 'dependence' to include an increasing number of drugs or "substances." The reasons for this expansion are a matter of debate. We tend to believe, like Goode[224], that it was primarily motivated by ideological reasons, or more specifically, by the wish "*to make sure that a discrediting label was attached to as many widely used drugs as possible* (p.47)." The expansion was achieved by substituting psychological and behavioral criteria for the pharmacological ones. A new term was introduced, **psychological dependence**, which described addiction that did not depend on withdrawal symptoms, in other words, addiction to drugs that by the classic pharmacological definition were not addictive drugs. This term was soon replaced by the more general **drug dependence**, which effectively blurred the distinction between physical and psychological dependence. This term was adopted in 1965 by the World Health Organization (WHO), which proposed that 'drug dependence' incorporate the conditions previously described as habituation and addiction[156]. In retrospect, this seems to have been the first step on the road to the current conceptual chaos in the field of addiction[594, A].

[A] The following paragraph by the eminent pharmacologist, Jaffe, provides a nice illustration of the current terminological chaos in the field of addiction: *"The term **addiction**, like the term **abuse**, has been used in so many ways that it can no longer be employed without further qualification or elaboration (...) In this chapter, the term **addiction** is used to connote a severe degree of **drug dependence** that is an extreme on a continuum of involvement with **drug use** (...) Anyone who is **addicted** would be considered **drug dependent** by the criteria described above. However, the term **addiction** cannot be used interchangeably with **physical dependence** as that term is used here. It is possible to be **physically dependent** on drugs without being **addicted** and, in some special circumstances, to be **addicted** without being **physically dependent** (...) The use of the terms **drug dependence**, to denote a behavioral syndrome, and **physical dependence**, to refer to biological changes that underlie withdrawal syndromes, causes confusion. To reduce some of this confusion, the term **neuroadaptation** has been proposed as a substitute for **physical dependence** (...)* (p. 523, bold added)[311]."

2.   BEHAVIORAL DEFINITIONS OF ADDICTION

The behavioral, as opposed to pharmacological, approach to addiction is exemplified by the diagnostic criteria for **Substance Dependence** in the current Diagnostic and Statistical Manual of Mental Disorders (DSM-IV)[10]. The DSM-IV defines Substance Dependence as a *"maladaptive pattern of substance use, leading to clinically significant impairment or distress."* This impairment or distress must be manifested by 3 of 7 criteria. Two of these criteria are tolerance and withdrawal; neither, however, is a necessary criterion for the disorder. Thus, according to the DSM-IV, one can be diagnosed with Substance Dependence if one takes a certain substance for a longer time than he or she intends to take it, makes unsuccessful efforts to cut down intake of the substance, and continues using the substance despite recurrent physical problems that have been exacerbated by the substance. In sharp contrast to the classic definition of addiction used by pharmacologists three decades ago, physical dependence is explicitly *not* a necessary criterion for a diagnosis of Substanc e Dependence in the DSM-IV. Therefore, while this definition shares the term 'dependence' with the classical pharmacological definition, the term does not actually *mean* the same in the two definitions. This has important consequences, as we shall discuss below.

3.   THE 1993 *WHO* DEFINITION OF DRUG DEPENDENCE

Most current definitions of drug dependence essentially adopted the behavioral definition of the term 'addiction.' This is illustrated by the most recent definition of addiction by the World Health Organization. In 1993, the WHO[711] defined 'drug dependence' (here used synonymously with addiction) *"as a cluster of physiological, behavioural and cognitive phenomena of variable intensity, in which the use of a psychoactive drug (or drugs) takes on high priority. The necessary descriptive characteristics are preoccupation with a desire to obtain and take the drug and persistent drug-seeking behaviour. Determinants and the problematic consequences of drug dependence may be biological, psychological or social, and usually interact* (p. 5)."

To the layman, "*a cluster of physiological, behavioural and cognitive phenomena of variable intensity*" (also used by the DSM-IV, albeit in different order) may sound very impressive. To the psychologist, this term means exactly the same as "behavior." All human efforts, from such basic ones as urinating to more complex ones as learning a language, are clusters of "*physiological, behavioural, and cognitive phenomena of variable intensity.*" Similarly, the sentence "*Determinants and the problematic consequences of drug dependence may be biological, psychological, or social, and usually interact*" applies to every conceivable human endeavor. In these respects there is no difference between drug dependence and the making of the first atomic bomb, eating of red meat (cholesterol!), bedwetting, or serving in the army. Moreover, whether consequences of drug consumption are psychologically or socially problematic or not depends to a large extent on the attitude of the society in which this behavior occurs. Coffee drinking could be made problematic by simply outlawing it. Thus, the wordy definition of the WHO[711] could be simplified by rephrasing it as "*a behaviour in which the use of a psychoactive drug (or drugs) takes on high priority. The necessary descriptive characteristics are preoccupation with a desire to obtain and take the drug and persistent drug-seeking behaviour.*"

When we examine both the DSM-IV and the WHO definitions, we find many common features. Most importantly, they both define addictive *behavior*, rather than addictive *drugs*. This approach opens a Pandora box of problems. The most serious problem is that the drugs are not assigned a clear *causal role* in the so-called addictive behavior. The behavior must involve the use of drugs, but neither definition requires that the drug have any causal role in maintaining the addiction. The definition of drug dependence, therefore, becomes a mere *description* of a habitual behavior, rather than a genuine *explanation* of it. This is difficult to see at first glance, because the word 'addiction' carries an *illusion* of an explanation: *Why* does the person in question continue to behave in a dysfunctional, self-defeating way? *Because* he or she is addicted. This has the sound, the structure of an explanation. But what does "addicted" mean in this context? It means nothing more than continuing to behave in a dysfunctional, self-defeating way. This is a completely circular account of the dysfunctional behavior. We must stress that such circularity does not characterize the original, pharmacological definition of addiction, in which the dysfunctional behavior is genuinely *explained* by the chemical properties of the addictive substance.

Another major problem, which we attend to next, is that addictive behavior as defined by the WHO and the DSM-IV is indistinguishable from habitual or compulsive behavior that has nothing to do with drugs. We explore this topic below, beginning with a general discussion of habit and continuing with a comparison of habits and addictions.

4.   THE NATURE OF HABITS

The term 'habit' entails a distinction between actions that result from conscious decision and actions that have been done many times and have become automatic[531]. This distinction was discussed more than a century ago by James[313], the great pioneer of scientific psychology: "*Any sequence of mental action which has frequently been repeated tends to perpetuate itself; so that we find ourselves automatically prompted to* think, feel, *or do what we have been before accustomed to think, feel, or do, under like circumstances, without any consciously formed* purpose, *or anticipation of results. (...) Habit simplifies the movements required to achieve a given result, makes them more accurate and diminishes fatigue* (p. 112)." A similar distinction, between *automatic* and *controlled* processes, was made by modern cognitive psychologists[e.g.,583,600]. Habits result from automatic processes that develop by repetition and are so well learned that no conscious processing is required. They are unintentional and typically set in motion by stimulus cues. They can go on simultaneously with other cognitive processes without any interference.

4.1   The Persistence of Habits

There is consensus among researchers, beginning with James himself[313], that the capacity to develop habits is adaptive to survival. It is hard to imagine life without habits. Habits enable humans and other organisms to selectively attend only to novel, complex and cognitively demanding tasks and to perform routine but necessary behaviors with minimal resources. If eating, walking, driving, tying shoe laces, brushing teeth etc. would have required our full attention, we would be severely restricted in performing other mental or physical activities at the same time.

Habits are a type of shortcut. They make life easier, if not possible, but every shortcut has a cost. The main cost of habits, as far as this book is concerned, is that they are resistant to change. Once behavior has been assigned to automatic processing, it is difficult to get it back under conscious control. When we perform something automatically, such as washing our hands, we are no longer aware of the steps that are involved in the process. Once these activities have become habits, they have functionally become a single unit of behavior which is no longer easy to modify. Moreover, whereas we are probably genetically prone to learn habits, we do not seem so prone to *un*learn them. This makes evolutionary sense. Learning new habits to free our attention to demanding tasks is essential to survival. This process is typically progressive: as we grow up, we develop more and more habits so that we can perform more and more routine activities without requiring costly attentional resources. The need to undo a habit is much less common. It arises only when environmental conditions change and the old habit is no longer advantageous, or, more relevant to our discussion, when we have unfortunately acquired a '*bad habit.*'

4.2   Good and Bad Habits

We commonly speak of 'good' and 'bad' habits. Good habits are those that promote efficient, functional, and healthy behavior. They are habits we are glad we have or, all too often, habits we wish we had. In fact, we often consciously attempt to develop good habits, that is, create useful automatic behavioral routines. Examples are putting our wallet and keys always in the same place as soon as we enter the house or checking the alarm clock before going to sleep. An exercise routine is a familiar example of a behavior that most of us strive to turn into a fixed habit, which will help insure its persistence[1]. Similarly, we attempt to instill in our children a variety of functional or socially acceptable good habits: wearing seatbelts, preparing homework before starting to play, eating with silverware, brushing teeth, or saying "thank you" regardless of how repulsive they think aunt Corey is and how cheap the gift she brought them.

Why do bad habits develop? The answer seems to be that the habit-learning mechanism is near-sighted. The capacity to make a routine behavior habitual is extremely useful; but the behaviors that are repeated until they become a habit may in fact be quite harmful in the long run. Our definition of a bad habit is simple: Bad habits are those we wish we did not have. What we consider bad habits may change, of course, depending on social norms and legal sanctions. Bad habits range from picking our nose through talking to ourselves to passing cars without looking at the rear mirror, and finally, to smoking cigarettes and using other harmful substances. We all have bad habits, and most of us are at war with one or more bad habits most of our lives. What we want to emphasize here is that bad habits are not necessarily more difficult to change than good ones. Habits are difficult to unlearn – this is why we talk of having to 'break' a habit. The reason we only run into problems with our bad habits is that we rarely try to change the good ones. We are frustrated with our bad habits and take our good ones for granted, thankless creatures that we are. But when we try to understand the difficulty of changing habits, we must be aware of the ubiquity of habits in all areas of our lives, good and bad ones alike.

5.   COMPULSIONS

Most of the literature on breaking habits involves what are commonly referred to as 'compulsive habits' or 'compulsions.' Compulsions are specific kinds of bad habits, consisting of dysfunctional, purposeful and repetitive behavioral routines. The word 'compulsion' reflects people's experience that they perform these habitual behaviors despite themselves; that they are *compelled* to perform them. The term 'compulsion' is usually attached to behaviors that carry short-term pleasure or relief of stress, but negative long-term consequences. Thus we talk about compulsive nail biting, scab picking, hair pulling, overeating, stealing, shopping, gambling, deviant or exaggerated sexual activity, etc. Clearly, not all gamblers, shoppers, or people who indulge in repetitive behaviors of this kind have a compulsion: the term 'compulsion' implies an attempt to resist the habit and/or a feeling of being controlled by the habit.

In the current psychiatric nosology, the term compulsion has become reserved to the defining symptoms of obsessive-compulsive disorder (OCD), in which the main symptoms are compulsive behaviors such as washing and checking, while other repetitive bad habits are classified in the diagnostic categories of impulse control, eating, or sexual disorders. In recent years, however, habit disorders have been re-united under the umbrella of "compulsive spectrum" or "obsessive-compulsive spectrum disorders," which is more in line with common usage[e.g.,55,285,731]. It is important to note that just like the distinction between a 'good' and a 'bad' habit, a habit is compulsive only to the extent that is recognized as excessive or dysfunctional by the individual with the habit, and is performed with a sense of resistance.

6.   HABIT CRAVING, WITHDRAWAL, AND RELAPSE

Compulsive habits are defined by a strong urge, or craving, to perform a certain act, such as pulling hair, binge eating, washing hands, stealing or masturbating. Performance of the act relieves the craving and may be accompanied by pleasure. Blockage of compulsive habits is accompanied by unpleasant symptoms, which always include increased craving to perform the blocked habitual activity, but may include also arousal, irritability, discomfort, insomnia, anxiety or depression. Such symptoms are commonly reported when obsessive-compulsive individuals, for example, try to resist a compulsion to wash their hands or check that the door is locked[402,511], when an individual with binge eating or bulimia tries to stay away from fattening but desirable food[362,415] or when a pathological gambler attempts to abstain from gambling[86,546].

In the latter study, for example[546], 222 pathological gamblers were queried regarding physical symptoms when attempting to slow down or stop gambling. Results were compared with the symptoms reported by 104 substance dependent individuals attempting to abstain from using their habitual substance. Sixty five percent of the gamblers experienced at least one of the following: insomnia, headaches, upset stomach, loss of appetite, physical weakness, heart racing, muscle aches, difficulty breathing, sweating, and chills. In fact, gamblers experienced *more* of these general withdrawal symptoms when attempting to stop gambling than did the substance dependent participants.

Overcoming bad or compulsive habits is an uphill battle and relapse rates are typically very high. A recent prospective study of OCD patients, most of whom were treated with appropriate antidepressant medications or behavior therapy, found a full remission rate of only 12 percent over two years. Partial remission rate was 47 percent, but of those who achieved full or partial remission during the two-year study, almost half (48 percent) relapsed by the end of the study[158]. Other studies have shown that when medication is discontinued, approximately 80 percent of successfully treated OCD patients relapse (reviewed by Ravizza et al.[517]).

A review of follow-up studies of patients with bulimia nervosa, which consists of compulsive binge eating and purging, reported that whereas approximately 50 percent of the patients achieved complete remission during the 5–10 years of follow-up, fully one-third relapsed by the end of the follow-up period[338]. The same rate of relapse was reported in another recent follow-up study of bulimia[275]. In a 2-year follow-up of exhibitionists, the rate of relapse was 75 percent[712]. A similar finding was reported in trichotillomania (compulsive hair pulling), where 8 of 12 patients who initially responded well to treatment relapsed during the follow-up period[375]. In a study of a comprehensive treatment program for gamblers, forty five percent reported partial or complete relapse at one-year follow-up[412]. Studies of Gamblers Anonymous, the most popular intervention for pathological gambling in the USA, suggest that only 8 percent of the attendants achieve a year of abstinence[487]. In a study of nail-biting, the relapse rate was 60–80 percent at an eight-week follow-up[287].

We can see, then, that habits, especially those we term 'bad' or 'compulsive,' share many attributes with drug addiction, including craving, persistence despite negative consequences, withdrawal symptoms and a tendency to relapse. Indeed, a critical consequence of the current behavioral definitions of addiction, as exemplified by the WHO and the DSM criteria, is that most of the criteria apply just as well to compulsive habits as they do to the use of substances. This equation of addiction with bad or compulsive habit is reflected in the proliferation of newly discovered addictions in recent years. *"Virtually anything that some people do with regularity, commitment, single-mindedness, or 'compulsion' has been called addiction. Persons are said to be addicted to television, to chocolate, to work, to sport, to candy, to gambling, to soft drinks, to coffee, to food, to exercise, to shopping, to sex, and to seemingly endless list of other consumable products and activities* (pp. 777–778)[8]." Thus, alcoholics have been joined by a multitude of other 'holics,' including chocoholics, workaholics, and sexaholics. This development has been reflected in the evolvement of the 12-step treatment programs for addictions. Initially conceived for alcohol (Alcoholics Anonymous, or AA) and later for narcotic addiction (NA), they now include not only Marijuana Anonymous and Cocaine Anonymous, but also Gamblers Anonymous, Overeaters Anonymous, Sexaholics Anonymous, Workaholics Anonymous, and even Debtors Anonymous (for people who have a compulsion to incur unsecured debts).

In summary, the new behavioral definitions of addictions describe a behavioral pattern, not properties of drugs. The patterns they describe, including craving, withdrawal symptoms and relapse, are indistinguishable from those that characterize compulsive habits. As a result, these definitions have promoted an equation between addiction and compulsive habits such as gambling, overworking and eating too much. The most critical problem for our purpose is that these definitions *do not specify what it means for a drug to be addictive*. Consequently, when we ask whether nicotine is addictive, we are left without criteria that would help us determine the answer. The fact that drugs are involved in a habit does not allow the inference that these drugs either *cause* or *maintain* the habit any more than hair causes trichotillomania, water causes hand-washing or store merchandise causes kleptomania. Nevertheless, as we discuss later in the book, exactly this kind of false inference has been made regarding the role of nicotine in smoking.

Chapter 3

HABITUAL DRUG USE

In the previous chapter we saw that once addiction is defined behaviorally, rather than by the chemical properties of drugs, it loses its specificity and becomes similar to other compulsive habits. We documented that compulsions, like drug addictions, continue in spite of harmful consequences and share with addictions the features of craving, withdrawal symptoms and tendency to relapse.

The similarity between drug addiction and habit is further complicated by the fact that most addictive drugs are used habitually, so that regular routines and rituals develop around the drug use. This point has been acknowledged in the DSM-IV[10]. In describing Opioid Dependence, for example, it notes that "*Persons with Opioid Dependence tend to develop such regular patterns of compulsive drug use...* (p. 248)."

The rituals that accompany the use of habitual drugs play an important part in maintaining the habit; in fact, eliminating them can sometimes cause an addiction to lose its appeal[478]. In heroin addiction, powerful components of the experience are not only the rite of self-injection but the overall lifestyle involved in the pursuit and use of the drug. Clinical experience indicates that drug users often crave not only the euphoria brought about by the drug but also the ritualistic procedure involved in its consumption. This might explain why pure heroin administered in a medical setting in Britain in the early 60s did not produce the satisfaction that individuals with heroin addiction receive from the adulterated street variety they were accustomed to self-administer[618].

It has long been reported that people with narcotic addiction can relieve their withdrawal symptoms by injecting sterile water[386]. Furthermore, when detoxified narcotic dependent individuals were asked to re-enact the injection procedure using saline solution, some of them reported mild opiate-like effects such as a "rush" and increased skin temperature[455]. Meyer and Mirin[420] allowed detoxified heroin dependent individuals access to heroin after pre-treating half of them with naltrexone (an opiate antagonist) and the other half with a placebo, using a double-blind design. Although the dose of naltrexone was adequate to block completely the effects of the subsequently injected heroin, there was a tendency for these participants to show weak but objectively measured opiate-like effects such as pupilary constriction and a reduction in respiratory rate. A similar finding was reported by Ternes and coauthors[650]. These and many other studies emphasize the important role of learning and specifically, habit formation, in determining craving, compulsion, relapse and other variables associated with habitual drug use[456,655].

The intimate relationships between addiction and compulsion in alcohol dependence were studied by Modell and his colleagues[426,427]. These researchers developed an instrument for measuring obsessive and compulsive characteristics of drinking-related thoughts and behaviors by modifying the Yale-Brown Obsessive-Compulsive Scale (Y-BOCS)[225]. Using the modified scale (Y-BOCS-hd), they showed similarities between obsessionality and compulsivity in OCD and in alcohol dependence. In the alcoholic population, subjectively rated craving for alcoholic beverages was correlated with alcohol-related thoughts and behaviors on the Y-BOCS-hd.

The same approach was applied to opiate addiction in a recent study[189]. Individuals with opiate dependence undergoing ambulatory treatment were interviewed about the importance of their opiate-use rituals, the severity of compulsivity and obsessionality in relation to their drug use, and their non-drug-related obsessive-compulsive symptoms. The results indicated that many opiate dependent individuals take their drugs in a ritualistic manner, and that the need for a fixed ritual is a major component in opiate dependence. The level of compulsivity and obsessionality in regard to opiate use was comparable to that found in OCD. In addition, based on established norms for OCD symptoms, the authors estimated that 11.4 percent of their sample would meet diagnostic criteria for OCD, a rate that is over 4 times the rate of OCD in the general population.

This research makes it clear that in habits that involve drugs, the effects of the drugs are not easily distinguished from the effects of the habits that form around its use. Both habit and physiological dependence can create craving, obsessions, persistent harmful behavior, general withdrawal symptoms, and relapse. Therefore, in a habit that involves psychoactive drugs, these effects cannot be attributed to the drug without independent evidence regarding the addictive qualities of the drug. We shall discuss what this evidence may consist of in the following chapters.

1. USE OF PSYCHOACTIVE DRUGS WITHOUT DEPENDENCE

We showed above that symptoms that are associated with addiction can occur in habits which do not involve drugs. We also showed that the effects of habits and drugs are confounded in the reality of habitual drug use, and cannot be attributed to the drug without independent evidence. To complete this discussion, we discuss the (possibly obvious) point that the involvement of psychoactive drugs in a habit does not in itself constitute addiction. We explicate this point by distinguishing several distinct patterns of habitual drug use. This distinction will serve to further illustrate the complexity of the subject matter, and more importantly, to clarify what kind of evidence is needed to imply nicotine as the chemical responsible for continued cigarette smoking.

1.1 The Ubiquity of Psychoactive Drugs

Nearly everyone uses one psychoactive drug or another. Most of us do so on a regular basis throughout most of our lives. In fact, in our classes at the university we often ask the students whether they use psychoactive drugs, and we have yet to encounter one who does not. Some use, on a daily basis, prescribed psychoactive drugs such as sedatives, anxiolytics or anti-depressants. Others use illicit drugs such as ecstasy, cocaine, heroin, or cannabis. However, such drug users are a minority. Most use psychoactive drugs that are common and legal, such as caffeine (in coffee and soft drinks like coca-cola), alcohol (in wine or beer) and the subject of this book – nicotine in cigarettes.

The same probably holds for all other countries in the world. Only for a minority of countries, however, systematic surveys assessing drug habits of the populations are available. We chose to rely on a recent survey performed in Amsterdam, Holland[561]. In this survey, over 4,000 respondents were asked to report which drug they had ever used, which they had used last year, and which they had used during the month preceding the survey. The results are shown in Table 3.1[B]. It is clear from this table that, apart from tobacco, alcohol, and cannabis (hashish and marijuana), drugs were tried by less than 8 percent of the sample, and less than 1 percent of the population of Amsterdam reported using these drugs recently (last month).

Table 3.1. Prevalence of drug use in Amsterdam in 1994. This Table and Table 2 are adapted with permission from the authors[561]. Values are the percentage of the total sample.

Drug	Lifetime	Last year	Last month
Tobacco	66.6	45.2	40.8
Alcohol	86.1	77.1	69.3
Cannabis	29.2	10.6	6.8
Cocaine	6.9	1.8	0.7
Amphetamines	4.7	0.5	0.3
Ecstasy	3.2	1.5	0.6
Hallucinogens	4.4	0.5	0.1
Inhalants	1.1	0.1	0.1
Opiates (all)	7.7	0.7	0.7

Table 3.1 shows that even without counting caffeine (which was not included in this survey), the vast majority of Dutch are psychoactive drug users. These drugs include alcohol and tobacco – two substances that involve health hazards about which the Dutch public has been informed for many years. Given that Dutchmen are as rational as the next human being, this demonstrates that drug use in spite of health hazards is normative. Most users would not be considered addicted – otherwise the term addiction would

[B] In Table 3.1 we did not include data on prescribed drugs (sedatives and hypnotics), as the fact that they are prescribed means that at least some of the people who take these drugs do not choose to consume them.

lose any specificity it still possesses – but some of them undoubtedly are. By which criteria can we distinguish between those who are addicted and majority who are not?

Table 3.2. Continuation rates in 1994 (in %)

Drug	Lifetime	Last year	Last month
Tobacco	100.0	67.5	61.4
Alcohol	100.0	89.6	80.5
Cannabis	100.0	36.1	23.3
Cocaine	100.0	25.6	10.8
Amphetamines	100.0	10.8	5.9
Ecstasy	100.0	46.0	20.4
Hallucinogens	100.0	11.5	2.6
Inhalants	100.0	21.3	10.6
Opiates (all)	100.0	27.6	8.6

Table 3.2 displays continuation data for those responders who had used psychoactive drugs at least once during their lifetime. These data show the vast majority of incidental users of illegal psychoactive substances do not become regular users. This is true for such drugs as hashish, cocaine, and amphetamines, but also for drugs which have a physical dependence potential such as opiates. Only a small minority of drug users (about 10 percent or less) continued to use cocaine, amphetamines, hallucinogens, inhalants, or opiates during the month preceding the survey. More continued in the case of hashish (23%) and ecstasy (20%). Lifetime frequency data obtained in this survey confirmed this pattern. By far, most of the drug users did not use the drug on more than 25 occasions. The noteworthy exceptions are alcohol and tobacco: more than 80 percent of the users used these substances on more than 25 occasions.

These observations are interesting in more than one respect. First, the potential for physical dependence of the illegal drugs does not predict their continuation rates. The continuation rate of cannabis is three times higher than that of opiates, although users are much more likely to develop physical dependence on the latter than on the former[311]. Hence, there must be other factors that determine why, after initial experimentation, a minority of users continues to take drugs.

Those factors are not necessarily the same for each drug. For example, Sandwijk and his coworkers[561] explained the relatively high continuation rate of ecstasy by its novelty. The drug hit the market a short time before the survey was conducted and therefore a larger proportion of the population "experimented" with it in the year and the month preceding the survey. This explanation would not hold, of course, for illegal "old-timers" such as cocaine, heroin, or cannabis.

A second point of interest is the high continuation rate for the legal drugs, alcohol and tobacco. The consumption of alcohol in Amsterdam is widespread (86% of the population used alcohol at least once during their life and 69% used alcohol during the month preceding the survey) although most drinkers (78%) consumed less than 3 glasses per day. The authors of the survey concluded, on the basis of these data, that "*Drinking alcohol is clearly an established habit in Amsterdam. (...) Nevertheless, consumption was usually rather moderate* (p. 125)[561]." Thus, whereas the use of alcohol takes on high priority in the Netherlands, the authors did not take this as evidence that many Dutch are alcoholics. It seems that there is more than one way to be a regular, and even an enthusiastic, consumer of alcohol – and not only in Holland.

1.2   Patterns of Substance Use

As we suspect some readers may know, "La Route des Vins" (the road of the wines) is not a street in Paris. It appears in the 1995 *Michelin Guide de Tourisme*[499] of the Upper Rhine ("*Rhin Superieur*, p. 143"), instructing wine aficionados how to reach the wine producers of the area. It is not unique: the route of the "*Vignoble et Eaux-vives*[498]" is another prime example of places where wine-lovers to whom the "*use of a psychoactive drug (or drugs) takes on high priority*" and who are preoccupied "*with a desire to obtain and take*" these drugs can indulge in "*persistent drug-seeking behavior,*" thus fulfilling all of the "*necessary descriptive characteristics*" of the 1993 WHO definition of drug dependence. The people whom we encountered on these roads, however, were no alcoholics, and drove their car (often full of wine boxes) with a steady hand. Most would agree that these wine enthusiasts should be differentiated from other Frenchmen, who, amidst many empty wine bottles use the warm grids over the Parisian Metro as their domicile on cold winter days.

In the previous chapter, we discussed the behavioral definitions for addiction or "drug dependence" proposed by the DSM-IV and the WHO. These definitions fail to distinguish clearly between the two types of drug users illustrated somewhat dramatically above. Both the wine connoisseur and the alcoholic may give high priority to the use of alcoholic drinks and go out of their way to purchase them. In fact, the craving of some wine-lovers for their "drug" is so great that they are willing to pay hundreds of dollars for a bottle of wine. An examination of the WHO and the DSM-IV criteria reveals that only the classic criteria for drug addiction – relating to physical dependence – distinguish these two patterns of drug use. Physical dependence, however, is no longer necessary for diagnosing drug dependence according to these two commonly accepted definitions.

In embarking on the subject of nicotine addiction, we must first clarify what nicotine addiction means. As we saw in this chapter and the previous one, the definition of drug addiction has changed over the years so it is no longer defined by physical dependence. Drug dependence, under the new definitions, is no more than a compulsive habit that involves drugs. The new definitions, unlike the classical pharmacological one, do not specify anything about the properties of the drug; specifically, they say nothing about how these properties may contribute to the initiation and maintenance of the habit. Unfortunately, as we showed in the previous chapter, habits involving drugs are very difficult to distinguish from habits that do not involve drugs, such as gambling, hair-pulling or exhibitionism, on the basis of behavior alone.

There are several classes of habits that are relevant to our discussion and should be clearly distinguished. The first class, which includes hair-pulling, kleptomania, pathological gambling, binge eating etc., comprises compulsive habits that do not involve psychoactive drugs. These habits are likely to have a biological basis (as do all common behaviors), so that their integrity depends on many biochemical mechanisms in the brain. But whatever purpose these habits serve and whatever pleasure and suffering they bring, they do not involve the consumption of psychoactive drugs. As we saw, these habits share essential features with drug addictions, including craving, persistence despite negative consequences, withdrawal symptoms such as irritability, anxiety, insomnia, and a high probability of relapse.

Habits that do involve consumption of psychoactive drugs can be divided into three classes. In the first class, the psychoactive properties of the drugs play only a minor role. Examples are moderate and discriminating consumption of wine and of coffee or tea. Although the psychoactive drugs contained in these beverages contribute to the user's pleasure, their contribution is a minor one. Typically, taste and smell are more rewarding than the psychoactive effects of the drug. This is evident from the "gourmet" cult that generally develops around these beverages. The wine connoisseur makes fine discriminations between different wines, and has preferences for very specific ones. He or she might settle at times for a basic table wine with dinner, but in the absence of wine would not resort to medicinal alcohol. It would be preposterous to argue that for such a person, wine is just a means of delivering alcohol to the bloodstream. This also holds for tea and coffee. While some people use coffee as a stimulant, for many others the psychoactive agent in the beverage may actually interfere with its consumption, as the success of decaffeinated coffee and tea testifies. For the distinguishing users, then, these habits seem to be little different from habits that do not involve drugs but provide sensory pleasure, like savoring cheeses or pastries.

In the second class of habits that involve psychoactive drugs, the drugs are important in sustaining the habit, yet even long-term use does not cause physical dependence. Thus, when the long-term consumption of these chemicals is ceased, no *drug-specific* withdrawal syndrome will appear. Of course "habit-withdrawal symptoms" may emerge, but these will resemble the distress following the interruption of habits that do not involve drugs, as detailed in the previous chapter. Typical drugs in this class are hashish, LSD, and mescaline.

Finally, the third type of drug-related habits are ones in which physical dependence develops. Cessation of drug consumption is followed by a withdrawal syndrome that involve both *drug-specific* withdrawal symptoms and general signs of distress such as follow the interruption of non-drug related habits. This is the only class that would have qualified for the label 'addiction' under the classic pharmacological definition.

2.   THE DRUG ATTRIBUTION BIAS

We showed earlier that pharmacologists had defined **addictive drugs** as having certain properties that, following long-term consumption, change the central nervous system in such a way that the organism is driven to continue consumption of the drug. The behavioral definition, on the other hand, concerns **addictive behavior**, which is characterized by craving, compulsivity, distress following cessation and a tendency to relapse. While every pharmacologist would consider these criteria *relevant* to drug addictions, they are not *exclusive* to habits that involve addictive chemicals. As we have demonstrated, these criteria apply to most compulsive habits, whether these habits involve drugs or not. Unlike the pharmacological definition, the behavioral definition does not require a *causal role* for the drug in maintaining the addictive behavior, which effectively makes the definition circular.

This circularity of the behavioral definition opens the door to a particular logical fallacy, which can be stated as follows: "Every drug that is addictive by pharmacological criteria produces a pattern of drug use that is addictive by behavioral criteria. A behavioral pattern that is addictive by behavioral criteria includes consumption of drug X. Therefore drug X is addictive by pharmacological criteria." When this syllogism is formulated explicitly, it is easy to see that it represents a logical fallacy. Nevertheless, we suggest that it represents a powerful attributional bias that has had a particularly detrimental effect on smoking research. This bias, which we shall refer to as **the drug attribution bias**, can be stated as follows: If a compulsive habit involves a psychoactive drug, observers will tend to attribute the habit to the drug *even if the drug has absolutely no causal role in motivating or maintaining the behavior*. For example, if we observed someone biting her nails compulsively, we would not assume that her behavior was caused by an addictive drug. If, however, we discover that during nail biting, some nail polish is ingested, we would tend to attribute the compulsive behavior to the nail polish even if, in reality, this "drug" has no role in causing the observed compulsion. In the next chapter, we will raise the possibility that the Surgeon General's declaration that nicotine is the addictive drug that causes smoking exemplifies this very seductive, but false, attributional bias.

Chapter 4

SMOKING DEFINED AS AN ADDICTION

1. THE SURGEON GENERAL REVIVES THE TERM 'ADDICTION'

By 1988, most of the medical literature had dropped the term 'addiction' like a hot potato. It was replaced by the term 'drug dependence,' which was not necessarily better defined, but was certainly more neutral. Only few researchers were still using the term 'addiction' and they, too, wished it were dropped[e.g.,311]. It is interesting, noting this trend, that the Surgeon General chose to revive 'addiction' from its timely death in his 1988 report on 'Nicotine Addiction[665].' This report states (p. 7) that *"The terms "drug addiction" and "drug dependence" are scientifically equivalent: both terms refer to the behavior of repetitively ingesting mood-altering substances by individuals. The term "drug dependence" has been increasingly adopted in the scientific and medical literature as a more technical term, whereas the term "drug addiction" continues to be used by NIDA and other organizations when it is important to provide information at a more general level. Throughout this Report, both terms are used and they are used synonymously."*

One can only guess what motivated the Surgeon General to re-introduce 'addiction' in his report on nicotine. Clearly, "drug dependence" and "drug addiction" are not really equivalent: The first is relatively free of moral and stigmatizing connotations, whereas the second is loaded with both. The argument that the two terms are "scientifically equivalent" because they both *"refer to the behavior of repetitively ingesting mood-altering substances by individuals"* is rather dubious. If this were the case, 'drug dependence' would be synonymous with a host of other terms, such as 'psychic dependence,' 'drug habituation,' or 'neuroadaptation,' all of which refer to the same behavior. Moreover, if terms become scientifically equivalent because they "refer" to the same behavior, then 'smoking,' 'injecting,' 'eating' and 'drinking' would also be scientifically equivalent and could be used synonymously, as they all refer to the self-administration of chemicals. Could the Surgeon General's decision to use the morally charged term 'addiction' have been tinged by non-scientific motivations?

The term 'addiction' was redefined by the 1988 report to mean something quite different from what it meant prior to 1988. To define nicotine as addictive, the Surgeon General could not use most previous definitions, not even his own from 1964[664], as according to these definitions nicotine would certainly *not* have been addictive. In 1964 he had defined "addiction" as requiring a well-defined state of intoxication, resulting in an impairment of judgement and/or cognition; a demonstration of tolerance, defined as a chronic need to increase an ingested dose to achieve the same biological and behavioral effect; and physical dependence as manifested by the appearance of adverse physical withdrawal symptoms upon cessation of use of the drug. In addition, an 'addict' was defined as suffering from occupational and social impairment as a result of his substance use. The substance tended to become the focal point of the addict's life, pushing other things such as job and family to the periphery[664]. Obviously, these criteria had to be changed drastically to accommodate nicotine addiction. In 1988, the Surgeon General[665] therefore redefined 'addiction' by proposing three sets of criteria. Below, we discuss these criteria in some detail. In the following chapters, we shall examine whether tobacco smoking meets the Surgeon General's revised criteria for drug addiction.

2. THE SURGEON GENERAL'S 1988 DEFINITION OF DRUG DEPENDENCE

According to the Surgeon General, the primary criteria of drug dependence are *"Highly controlled or compulsive use," "Psychoactive effects,"* and *"Drug-reinforced behavior."* The Report further states: *"The primary criteria listed above are sufficient to define drug dependence. Highly controlled or compulsive use indicates that drug-seeking and drug-taking behavior is driven by strong, often irresistible urges. It can persist despite a desire to quit or even repeated attempts to quit. Such behavior is also referred to as "habitual" behavior. To distinguish drug dependence from habitual behaviors not involving drugs, it must be demonstrated that a drug with psychoactive (mood-altering) effects in the brain enters the blood-stream. Furthermore, drug dependence is defined by the occurrence of drug-motivated behavior; therefore the psychoactive chemical must be capable of functioning as a reinforcer that can directly strengthen behavior leading to further drug ingestion* (p. 8)[665]*."*

The explanatory section strengthens the impression that 'addiction' was redefined to accommodate nicotine, which could not be defined as addictive by the criteria that have been used for other drugs such as opiates, barbiturates, or alcohol. The phrase *"to distinguish drug dependence from habitual behaviors not involving drugs"* shows that the Surgeon General was reluctant to allow for the third possibility we have discussed earlier, namely that drugs can be involved in a habit without the user becoming dependent on them. This redefinition thus paves the way to labeling any habit which involves a psychoactive drug as drug-dependence or addiction. This aim is also served by the specification that the three primary criteria are sufficient to define drug dependence, so that the classic criteria of physical dependence and tolerance, which are clearly met by opiates and alcohol but are quite problematic in the case of nicotine, are no longer required.

As we discussed in the previous chapters, the behavioral definitions of addiction, such as those of the DSM-IV[10] and the WHO[711], concern addictive behavior rather than addictive drugs. They describe a compulsive habit in which a drug is involved, but in contrast to the classic definitions of addiction, say nothing about the properties of the drug that presumably maintains the habit. As such, they cannot be used to define nicotine, or any other drug, as addictive. The Surgeon General seems to have recognized this inherent flaw in the behavioral definitions of addiction, which would not have allowed him to declare nicotine the addictive drug that maintains the smoking habit. Accordingly, his definition, though it still concerns behaviors rather than drugs, does specify two requirements regarding the drug itself: The drug must have psychoactive effects and it must be capable of directly reinforcing behavior.

A close inspection, however, reveals that the first criterion, namely that the drug have psychoactive effects, leaves much to be desired. In the first place, psychoactivity means completely different things for different drugs. The psychoactivity of LSD is characterized by hallucinations and reality distortion, whereas alcohol's psychoactive effects involve interference with the ability to concentrate, to speak clearly, to walk and to perform sexually. Second, psychoactivity is very weakly related to drug dependence. Some medications on which the user is dependent in the strongest sense of the word – without it he or she might die – are not known to have significant psychoactive effects. Insulin preserves the life of people with diabetes mellitus, and alpha-blockers reduce high blood pressure. Is there doubt that people who use these medications are at least as drug-dependent – scientifically if not morally – as are cigarette smokers? Finally, the Surgeon General does not specify that the psychoactive effects are the reason for which the drug is taken. In fact, he does not specify that these effects must be pleasant, or desirable, or in any way promote the use of the drug. Again, we believe this was not merely an oversight. A clearer statement of the causal relationship between psychoactive effects and addiction would have made it much more difficult to make the case for nicotine addiction, as we shall show in later chapters.

In contrast to the authors of the WHO and the DSM IV definitions, the Surgeon General recognized that to justify the diagnosis of addiction or drug-dependence, the drug must have a causal role in maintaining the drug-related habit. He states that *"drug dependence is defined by the occurrence of drug-motivated behavior; therefore the psychoactive chemical must be capable of functioning as a reinforcer that can directly strengthen behavior leading to further drug ingestion* (p. 8)." Unlike psychoactivity, this criterion is neither trivial nor irrelevant; in fact, much of the rest of this book is dedicated to reviewing the research on the reinforcing properties of nicotine. Before proceeding to explore this issue, however, we examine the remaining criteria for drug addiction proposed by the Surgeon General. Our purpose in so doing is to demonstrate that none of these criteria are capable of distinguishing drug-related from other compulsive habits; therefore, they have no bearing on the question of nicotine addiction.

3. PRIMARY CRITERIA

3.1 Highly Controlled or Compulsive Use

"Highly controlled or compulsive use indicates that drug-seeking and drug-taking behavior is driven by strong, often irresistible urges. It can persist despite a desire to quit or even repeated attempts to quit. Such behavior is also referred to as "habitual" behavior" (p. 7–8)."

Even to the layperson, this criterion of drug dependence would seem very weak. Its weakness is made especially evident in the last sentence, which clarifies that all this criterion means is that drug dependence must be a habit. Many unwanted behaviors fit the description that they are "driven by strong, often irresistible urges" and persist despite a desire or attempts to quit. Compulsive hand washing, for example, clearly fits this criterion, yet has nothing to do with drugs or dependence on any chemical. So are most other 'compulsive spectrum disorders' such as binge eating, pathological gambling, compulsive nail biting, kleptomania, trichotillomania, compulsive masturbation, or exhibitionism. All these are behaviors that are harmful to the individual performing them, at least in the long run, but that he or she feels helpless to control. Hence, while the compulsive nature of the behavior may be justified as a necessary criterion of drug dependence, it has no relevance for distinguishing drug dependence from other harmful habits.

In addition to the primary criteria, the Surgeon General lists additional criteria that are *"often used to characterize drug dependence* (p. 8)." None of these additional criteria, as shown below, has any value in distinguishing drug dependence from other harmful habits, specifically those comprising the 'compulsive spectrum' of behaviors.

4.   SECONDARY CRITERIA

4.1   The Behavior May Develop into Regular Temporal and Physical Patterns of Use (Repetitive and Stereotypic)

This clearly fits most of the compulsive spectrum behaviors. People with obsessive-compulsive disorder (OCD) display repetitive, stereotypic behavior in performing their rituals; in fact, compulsions are defined in the DSM IV as repetitive and stereotypic[10]. A person with bulimia will typically perform her bingeing at a particular time of the day, in the same location, with certain foods; she will then proceed to vomit or otherwise purge in a fixed routine. People with trichotillomania will tend to pull out hair from specific locations in the body, on a particular sofa, at a certain time of the day; and so on. Furthermore, stereotypic "drug use" is common in the absence of any addiction.   Many people have a fixed ritual of coffee preparation and consumption: They buy a specific variety of the "drug" at a particular store, store it in a special container, grind it fresh each morning, prepare it in a fixed and meticulous fashion, and drink it with a their favorite cup – behaviors that are very similar to those recently reported with heroin addicts[189].

4.2   Drug Use May Persist Despite Adverse Physical, Psychological or Social Consequences

Take the words "drug use" out, and you can substitute any bad habit: overeating, nail-biting, gambling, exhibitionism, kleptomania.

4.3   Quitting Episodes Are Often Followed by Resumption of Drug Use (Relapse)

As we showed above, bad habits are notoriously difficult to break. Again, in the above sentence, "drug use" can be replaced with "gambling," "bingeing and purging," or just "bad habit" with no ill effects to its validity.

We discuss this issue again in Chapter 10, where we compare the relapse rates associated with overeating to those associated with smoking cessation.

4.4 Urges (Cravings) to Use the Drug May Be Recurrent and Persistent, Especially During Drug Abstinence

The term 'craving' has been much criticized as a criterion of drug addiction[683]. As we showed earlier, most compulsive spectrum disorders are characterized by strong urges to perform the habit. Obsessions in OCD, which are characterized in the DSM IV as *"recurrent and persistent[10]"* are often experienced as urges to perform the compulsive rituals. Similarly, sexual paraphilias are typically preceded by urges to perform the forbidden sexual act, overeating by urges to eat, and so forth. These urges are experienced as stronger the more the person tries to resist acting on them or is blocked from performing them. In contrast, physical dependence on alcohol is characterized by a dysphoric, drug-specific withdrawal syndrome that lends a different meaning to the word 'craving.' In this regard, Kozlowski and Wilkinson[356] asked: *"Are desires for alcohol, tobacco, and other drugs different? If yes, in what ways do they differ? Is it simply that the desires are the same but the physiological correlates are different?* (p. 490)" Hughes[291], who also pointed to the many different connotations of the term 'craving' stated: *"In summary, I believe that, at present, the variety of meanings for the construct of craving precludes its utility* (p. 38)."

5. TERTIARY CRITERIA

5.1 Dependence-Producing Drugs Often Produce: Tolerance, Physical Dependence, and Pleasant (Euphoriant) Effects

Whereas these used to be the primary criteria for drug addiction for many decades, as discussed earlier, the Surgeon General delegated them to the very end of his list of criteria. This change, we believe, is no accident: As we aim to show in the remainder of the book, had these classic criteria retained their primary status, it would be extremely difficult to justify labeling nicotine an addictive drug. Furthermore, the criterion is worded so that tolerance, physical dependence and pleasant effects *need not be causally related* to the addiction. In genuinely addictive psychoactive substances, such as heroine, tolerance occurs to the *euphoric* (pleasant) effects of those drugs, and the withdrawal syndrome following abstinence from these drugs is strongly *dysphoric*, so both effects *cause* continued use. As he did for psychoactive effects as one of the primary criteria, the Surgeon General waived the need for proving a causal relationship between tolerance and physical dependence on the one hand, and mood changes induced by drugs or by drug abstinence, on the other.

6.   THE SURGEON GENERAL'S CONCLUSIONS REGARDING NICOTINE ADDICTION

The three Major Conclusions of the Report of the Surgeon General[665] on nicotine addiction (p. 9) are:

> *"1. Cigarettes and other forms of tobacco are addicting*
>
> *2. Nicotine is the drug in tobacco that causes addiction*
>
> *3. The pharmacologic and behavioral processes that determine tobacco addiction are similar to those that determine addiction to drugs such as heroin and cocaine."*

When these conclusions were published, not everyone agreed that they were empirically justified. One of their sharpest critics was Warburton, a well-known smoking researcher, who had the following to say about the first two conclusions: *"Of course, nicotine use can be called an "addiction;" someone, like the Surgeon General, just has to say it is. As Lewis Carroll wrote:*

"When I use a word", Humpty Dumpty said in rather a scornful tone, "it means just what I choose it to mean – neither more nor less"

"The question is," said Alice, "whether you can make words mean so many different things."

"The question is," said Humpty Dumpty, "which is to be master – that's all".

However, the most important measure for a scientific claim is experimental verification, not political pronouncements, however masterful (p. 169)[683]."

7. EXPLORING THE EMPIRICAL BASIS FOR NICOTINE ADDICTION

The main goal of this book is to examine the empirical evidence for nicotine addiction. As suggested above, in habits that include known psychoactive drugs, there is a tendency to attribute the habit to the drug even if no causal role for the drug has been demonstrated. This 'drug attribution bias' might lead to implicating nicotine as the cause of the smoking habit in the absence of any empirical basis. Even more importantly, as we shall discuss in the final chapter of the book, debates about drug use and its implications for society are not limited to the academic world. Non-academic authorities, such as government agencies, legislators, moral pressure groups, the tobacco industry and others contribute to the debate and turn it from a scientific discussion of evidence to an emotional exchange where fears, wishful thinking, and propaganda contribute as much, and sometimes even more, than facts. It is not inconceivable, in that context, that the Surgeon General was interested in portraying smoking as an addiction and nicotine as an addictive substance, a motivation which might lead to a biased interpretation and weighing of research results.

Such a bias may be reflected in the third conclusion of the Surgeon General (see above), which Warburton[683] saw as no more than "*an argument by analogy. Argument by analogy may be used to suggest a conclusion, but it cannot establish it. The force of the argument by analogy depends upon the resemblance of the defining properties of X and Y. It only needs Y to possess some property that X does not, for the analogy to be unsound and the conclusion fallacious, no matter how many properties X and Y have in common* (p. 166)." Indeed, there is a vast literature on the different pharmacological and behavioral effects of cocaine and heroin, especially when it comes to the addictive properties of these chemicals. If these drugs are entirely different from each other, how can nicotine resemble both of them? The claim for similarity (see Chapter 13) requires a selective process of stressing similarities (even if they are not relevant to mechanisms of addiction) while, at the same time, de-emphasizing or ignoring the differences.

What, then, would constitute scientific evidence, rather than "*political pronouncements, however masterful*" for nicotine addiction? In previous chapters we showed that the current definitions of addiction, in contrast to the classical pharmacological ones, define addictive behavior rather than addictive drugs. The Surgeon General's definition of drug addiction (or dependence) generally follows the same tradition, in that one of the primary criteria and all of the secondary criteria are behavioral. Unlike other behavioral definitions, however, this definition does require that the drug should possess psychoactive effects and reinforcing properties, which are two of the primary criteria for addiction (other properties of the drug, such as physical dependence and tolerance, are not required). At the same time, the drug's psychoactive effects are not specified, and are not causally related to its "*highly controlled or compulsive use,*" "*stereotypic patterns of use,*" or "*use despite harmful effects.*" Similarly, nothing about the drug itself is necessarily related to "*relapse following abstinence*" and "*recurrent drug cravings.*" As we showed in the previous chapters, this is not a trivial oversight: compulsive and stereotypic behavior, craving and relapse can all occur in the absence of any drug. The only place in the definition where a causal relationship between the drug and the behavior is stated is the requirement that the drug should be capable of directly reinforcing behavior, which presumably would lead to continued use. Consequently, testing the nicotine addiction hypothesis essentially reduces to testing whether nicotine is reinforcing. It is not surprising, therefore, that a huge number of studies have attempted to establish the reinforcing properties of nicotine in animals and humans.

Chapter 5

NICOTINE REINFORCEMENT IN ANIMALS: THEORETICAL CONSIDERATIONS

Our examination of the Surgeon General's primary criteria for drug addiction, by which nicotine was declared an addictive drug, revealed that they do not include the classic requirements of drug-specific withdrawal symptoms or tolerance. The only causal role required for the drug in maintaining the habit was that "*the psychoactive chemical must be capable of functioning as a reinforcer that can directly strengthen behavior leading to further drug ingestion* (p. 8)[665]." Consequently, we shall dedicate the next four chapters to an exploration of the reinforcing properties of nicotine. We begin with a theoretical exposition of reinforcement and the related learning principles, followed by a description of self-administration procedures, based on these principles, for assessing the reinforcing value of drugs. We then proceed to discuss of what constitutes evidence for establishing the reinforcing properties of drugs and particularly nicotine, in self-administration procedures.

1.   OPERANT REINFORCERS

The term 'reinforcer' is derived from animal learning theory, and plays a central role in the paradigm of 'operant' or 'instrumental' conditioning[611]. In this context, a reinforcer is an event which, when contingent upon given behavior, increases the probability and the frequency that this behavior will be repeated.

The effects of reinforcers in the laboratory are typically tested on rats in a box designed by Skinner and known as an 'operant chamber.' It normally contains a lever, or bar, which the animal can press. Rats press the lever the first time by chance, often by leaning on it while exploring their new environment. Pressing the lever can produce two kinds of consequences. The first are rewarding, or pleasurable, effects, and are called **positive reinforcers**. For example, a food pellet may fall into the feeder. The animal will eat the pellet and, after a while, press again. Another food pellet will appear. Within a short time, the animal will learn the connection between the lever press and the food, and will continue to press for as long as it is hungry.

In the same manner, rats can be trained to press a lever to stop an aversive stimulus, such as a painful electrical shock to their feet. If animals learn to press the lever in order to avoid an event, such events are called **negative reinforcers**. The relationship between the administration of positive or negative reinforcements and lever pressing can be manipulated by the investigator and is referred to as a **schedule of reinforcement**. Reinforcements in the studies we shall discuss are typically delivered in a **fixed ratio** of bar presses. If they are delivered every time the animal presses the bar, the ratio is referred to as 'Fixed Ratio 1 (FR1);' if at every other time, 'Fixed Ratio 2 (FR2),' etc.

1.1   Drugs as Positive Operant Reinforcers: The Self-Administration Paradigm

The positive reinforcing value of drugs for animals can be tested, in principle, by reversing the logic of operant reinforcement procedures. When a scientist trains a rat to press the lever for food, he or she has *a priori* knowledge that food is rewarding to rats. In the case of drugs, such prior knowledge is absent; instead, what the scientist wants to learn by using a drug in this paradigm is *whether* a given drug has reinforcing properties. The logic is that *if* rats will press a lever to receive a drug, this drug must be reinforcing to rats. Pressing a lever for a drug is referred to as **drug self-administration**, and the procedure is considered crucial for testing the reinforcing properties of drugs.

In a typical self-administration procedure, an intravenous tube is implanted in the rat, which is then placed in an operant chamber. The intravenous tube is attached to a syringe in a pump that will automatically activate the plunger of the syringe whenever the lever is pressed, and deliver a predetermined amount of the drug. Technically, this is a simple procedure; but the interpretation of its results is far from straightforward.

Let us consider a hypothetical study in which rats receive intravenous injections of heroin solution every time they press the lever. Few people will doubt that heroin is highly addictive by any criterion. Most rats will slowly learn to press the lever repeatedly and, after many trials, will self-administer heroin in a regular way, as other rats will press for food reward. Furthermore, rats receiving heroin will press the lever more frequently than rats receiving intravenous injections of water. Do these results enable us to conclude that heroin is a positive reinforcer for the rat, i.e., that it increases behavior because it is pleasurable?

Not necessarily. There are other possible explanations. For one, it is often difficult to discern whether, in a given situation, a drug acts as a positive or a negative reinforcer, or both. Heroin, as is well known, produces physical dependence, meaning that cessation after long-term use produces highly unpleasant withdrawal symptoms. To repeat Shuster's phrase, "*the addicted animal seems to be 'well' while intoxicated but becomes ill when the poison is removed*[606]." As this syndrome can be prevented, or stopped, by taking more heroin, the drug acts as a *negative* reinforcer: animals will maintain heroin self-administration in order to stop the presumably aversive effects of withdrawal. Hence, in the absence of other evidence, the demonstration that rats can be trained in the operant chamber to self-administer heroin is not sufficient proof for either the positive or the negative reinforcing properties of this substance.

Matters are further complicated by the fact that it is often difficult to train rats to self-administer drugs in the operant chamber. In many studies, therefore, rats are initially trained to press a lever for food reward, which they readily do. When they have learned to consistently press the lever for food, the food pellet is replaced with an intravenous injection of a drug. Thus, these experiments do not test whether rats are willing to *initiate* lever pressing for a drug, but rather whether the drug can *maintain* the lever pressing that had been acquired with food reward. The problem with this procedure is that a drug can maintain lever pressing in this procedure even if, inherently, it produces neither reward (positive reinforcement) nor physical dependence (negative reinforcement). Specifically, a drug can become a **secondary reinforcer** by classical conditioning processes.

2.   PRIMARY AND SECONDARY REINFORCERS

In the famous experiments of Pavlov[477], dogs began to salivate at the sound of a bell after it was paired repeatedly with administration of meat powder. In this procedure, meat powder was not an operant reinforcer, as it was not contingent on the dogs' behavior. It was *always* administered following the sounding of the bell, whether or not the dogs salivated after hearing the bell. Therefore, it was not a response that was learned, but an association between two stimuli. A formerly neutral event (the sound of the bell) acquired, by association with meat powder, stimulus properties it did not have before. Meat powder is an **unconditioned stimulus** for dogs – it produces salivation inherently, without learning. The sound of a bell, in contrast, is a **conditioned stimulus** in this paradigm: it produces salivation by the association of its sound with meat powder. Within the instrumental conditioning framework, unconditioned stimuli are termed **primary reinforcers**, meaning that their reinforcing properties are inherent, whereas conditioned stimuli are termed **secondary reinforcers** (for review, see Domjan and Burkhard[146]). In the operant chamber, certain secondary reinforcers may be just as effective in training rats as some primary reinforcers. Secondary reinforcers are also effective rewards for humans. Money, for example, is a strong positive reinforcer for humans. However, unlike primary reinforcers like food, the reinforcing properties of money are learned – money has no reinforcing properties for babies or for adults in a culture that does not use it.

In the same manner, aversive stimuli can be paired with neutral stimuli and become secondary *negative* reinforcers. As Pavlov has demonstrated, if the sound of a bell is paired with a painful electrical shock to the foot, dogs will learn to lift their paw, whine, and show other signs of discomfort at the sound of the bell. In an instrumental learning paradigm, if dogs have previously learned to avoid electric shock by jumping over a barrier, they will now do so in response to the sound of the bell. The sound of the bell, which had been paired with a primary negative reinforcer (shock to the foot), becomes a secondary negative reinforcer.

2.1   Drugs as Secondary Reinforcers

When animals are thoroughly trained to press a lever for food reward, the lever itself may acquire secondary reinforcing properties. This becomes apparent when food reinforcement is discontinued: In spite of the lack of reward, animals will press the lever frequently before the response is finally extinguished. Furthermore, the lever will retain its reinforcing properties for a considerable length of time. If the animals are returned to the Skinner box several days following extinction, they will start to press the lever immediately. Thus, when drugs are substituted for food following the acquisition of lever pressing, drug injections may acquire reinforcing properties by being paired with the lever press[C].

Summing up our discussion so far, we have seen that drugs can maintain self-administration without being rewarding, by at least two mechanisms. First, repeated injections may produce physical dependence, and a dysphoric withdrawal syndrome may give rise to negatively reinforcing properties the drug did not initially possess. Second, and more important in the case of nicotine, a drug may acquire reinforcing properties by classical conditioning to primary or even secondary reinforcers.

3.   CONFOUNDING FACTORS IN STUDYING THE REINFORCING PROPERTIES OF DRUGS

Learning, as we have stated before, is a highly complicated behavior. It depends not only on motivational factors, such as reinforcement, but also on an appropriate state of arousal. In addition, learning requires that the animal remember the event. Specifically, in order for learning to occur, the

---

[C] This mechanism explains, at least in part, the ubiquity of 'placebo' effects. When animals or humans expect a certain effect from a drug (pleasure, analgesia, or anything else) a neutral drug will produce the anticipated effect. Placebo effects are well known and can be extremely powerful[e.g.,95,178,243,337,688,694,713]. In the context of nicotine-related experiments, the possible presence of placebo effects complicates the interpretation of the results (see Chapter 11).

encoding, consolidation and *retrieval* of the reinforcer, the behavior, and its consequences must take place.

In humans, as in rats, motivation, arousal, learning, and memory are mediated by neurons in the central nervous system. Psychoactive drugs act on various neurotransmitters that conduct the information to neurons in the brain. Heroin, for example, acts on endorphin receptors, whereas cocaine and amphetamine act on dopamine and noradrenaline receptors.

Any given neurotransmitter can be involved in the regulation of many brain functions. For example, there is considerable evidence that the endorphins are involved in pain perception, feeding, temperature regulation and sexual behavior. Heroin mimics the effects of the endorphins. When humans self-administer heroin, or any other drug, they do so *systemically* – to the entire system. The drug circulates throughout the body, reaching every site in the central nervous system. Consequently, heroin will affect all functions in which endorphins play a role. Some of these functions are motivational, which may explain the rewarding effects of heroin. But other functions may concern one or more phases of learning, memory consolidation or retrieval.

Consider a study in which rats are trained to press a lever to obtain food. Once they have learned this behavior thoroughly, the researcher stops reinforcing their behavior by withholding the food reward. At this stage, extinction should occur: The animals must learn that pressing the lever is no longer followed by a reward, and that they can therefore stop pressing. However, in this study the animals are now injected with a drug that prevents memory consolidation. As a result, the rats may fail to acquire extinction and will continue to press the lever and self-administer the drug *even if it does not have any reinforcing properties*.

In the same vein, a memory enhancing drug, mimicking the action of another neurotransmitter, could facilitate learning without necessarily providing reinforcement for that learning. Indeed, several animal experiments in which drugs were delivered into discrete brain areas have demonstrated that drugs can inhibit or enhance memory processes (for review, see White[706]). It is possible, with appropriate experimental controls, to distinguish between motivational and other learning-related effects. As we shall see later, however, such controls were rarely employed when the reinforcing properties of nicotine were investigated.

The systemic effects of certain drugs, such as cocaine and amphetamines, commonly lead to increased arousal and a corresponding increase in spontaneous or learned behaviors. Other drugs, such as heroin and barbiturates (at least at high doses), tend to decrease arousal and behavior. It is no accident that in the jargon of users amphetamine is called 'speed' and barbiturates 'downers,' or that morphine received it name from Morpheus, the Greek god of dreams and sleep. As we will show in our discussion of electrical self-stimulation (see Chapter 7), the effects of drugs on arousal, like their effects on memory, may confound the interpretation of experimental results.

In conclusion, the Surgeon General's requirement that "*the psychoactive chemical must be capable of functioning as a reinforcer that can directly strengthen behavior leading to further drug ingestion* (p. 8)[665]" cannot be met simply by showing that the drug maintains self-administration. The research must also establish (1) that the drug did not acquire its reinforcing properties as a secondary reinforcer, and (2) that the drug does not maintain self-administration by affecting memory or arousal.

4.   SPECIFIC PROBLEMS IN STUDYING NICOTINE SELF-ADMINISTRATION IN ANIMALS

The discussion above shows that self-administration is not sufficient to demonstrate unequivocally that a drug is a primary reinforcer for animals. Therefore, researchers aiming to establish the reinforcing value of drugs must employ controls that will allow them to rule out alternative explanations of their results. In addition to the general requirements specified above, nicotine presents unique problems that must be addressed by studies that investigate whether or not it is a reinforcer. To begin with, there are strong indications that nicotine increases response rate regardless of whether or not drug-delivery is contingent on responses. Below, we discuss several mechanisms that can produce this phenomenon.

4.1   Nicotine Produces General Activation and Stimulates Ongoing Behavior

Nicotine, at low doses, increases overall activity in rats. At higher doses, nicotine initially depresses and then re-activates ongoing behavior[16,35,68,98,99,102,117,118,196,248,260,322,361,433,438,441,457,519,521,544,571,574,579,604,633,695]. Tolerance of the depressant effect occurs and, subsequently, the stimulant action of nicotine becomes more pronounced with repeated administration [e.g.,99,102,695]. In all of the above experiments nicotine increased spontaneous locomotion. The nicotine antagonist mecamylamine blocks both the depressant and the stimulant effects, indicating that both are produced by nicotinic receptors[99,102].

Increased activation can affect various responses made by animals, including lever pressing. Clarke and Kumar[101] tested the effects of nicotine in rats trained to shuttle (move from one part of a shuttlebox to the other) for rewarding electrical brain stimulation. They noted that with repeated daily nicotine injections, a marked, dose-dependent, stimulant effect emerged – even when brain stimulation was turned off. These results were replicated by the authors themselves and by another team[100,571]. Others have shown that nicotine activates other operant behaviors such as lever pressing for food[218,368,432,505,705] or for water[212].

In summary, nicotine in low doses or in repeated administration stimulates ongoing behavior. If an animal happens to be walking, shuttling, or pressing a lever, nicotine will make it walk, shuttle, or press even more. As Wise and Bozarth[720] pointed out, when the animal presses a lever to self-administer nicotine, it may enter a positive feedback loop in which nicotine activates further pressing for nicotine, not because of its reinforcing properties, but because of its activating ones.

This possibility gains credence from the finding that rats pressing a lever for intravenous nicotine also pressed more on a second lever, which had no reinforcing consequences[122]. This is a finding that highlights the non-specific activating effect of nicotine in self-administration studies. Similarly, the observation that selective dopamine antagonists blocked both nicotine-induced locomotion and nicotine self-administration[117] suggests that these antagonists reduce the non-specific stimulant properties of nicotine.

Thus, the observation that nicotine stimulates any ongoing behavior, a property that may well play a major role in nicotine self-administration, is well established. It is therefore intriguing that the vast majority of studies on nicotine self-administration, as we shall see in the next chapter, did not make any attempt to control for it.

4.2   Food Deprivation Induces Non-Specific Activation

In many studies of nicotine self-administration, the rats are food deprived before the start of the conditioning procedure[e.g.,115,148]. The reason for this is simple: In contrast to the case with powerfully reinforcing drugs such as morphine, heroin and cocaine[60,408,451,674,721], rats that are not hungry are annoyingly reluctant to self-administer nicotine[e.g.,689]. But whereas food deprivation is often essential to get the rats to use nicotine, it introduces another confounding factor in these studies: Hunger activates behavior in rats, a phenomenon just as well-documented as the stimulating effect of nicotine. Food-restriction causes a remarkable increase in the use of activity-wheels and may lead to the cessation of the estrous cycle in females, loss of body weight, and even self-starvation[e.g.,331,376,377,547,548,563,622,624,687,725], a phenomenon that has been proposed as an animal model of anorexia nervosa[15,133,134,135,496]. Such general activation may well increase the rate of lever pressing in self-administration studies, an effect that is liable to be falsely attributed to the reinforcing properties of nicotine.

4.3   Nicotine Interferes with Extinction by Preserving Memory

There is another explanation for the self-administration of nicotine by animals, which has nothing to do with its providing reinforcement contingent upon the response. This explanation is relevant to those paradigms where animals are pre-trained to self-administer known reinforcing agents such as food, water, or other drugs such as cocaine, and are subsequently switched to nicotine[e.g.,115,148,527,562,636]. By these training procedures the animals "come to expect" a given reinforcer. Remarkably, in none of the self-administration studies reviewed here were the animals subjected to an adequate extinction procedure, where the original reinforcement was withheld so that the animal learned not to expect a reinforcing event and stopped pressing. Consequently, for at least the first 5–10 nicotine self-administration sessions, the results are confounded: They reflect not only nicotine-reinforced pressing, but also the residual effects of the original reinforcer. In subsequent sessions, the animals are presur. d to have "forgotten" the original reinforcer, so that continued lever pressing now reflects the reinforcing power of nicotine. This presumption, however, is problematic.

Nicotine, as has been demonstrated in dozens of experimental studies, has a positive effect on cognitive processing in normal humans and animals[for review, see 378,382,684,686] as well as in Alzheimer's patients[e.g.,324,528,715]. Some of the improvement may be due to increased arousal but, particularly in animals, nicotine and its agonists seem to have specific effects on working memory[382]. With nicotinic agonists, *"memory is facilitated to such a degree that animals 'fail' to forget their previous responses* (p. 219)[382]."

In the procedure described above, animals that have been trained to press a lever for food or cocaine undergo extinction under the influence of nicotine. Since nicotine preserves their memory of food or cocaine reinforcement and of their own response, their acquired responses may extinguish more slowly than in animals that are not injected with nicotine. Thus, as White[706] suggested, the crucial factor that sustains response in these experimental paradigms may be nicotine's effect on learning processes rather than its reinforcing properties.

5. CONCLUSIONS

The discussion in this chapter has focused on theoretical issues involved in demonstrating the reinforcing properties of nicotine in self-administration studies. We have shown that careful controls must be employed in such studies, to insure that self-administration can be attributed with confidence to the reinforcing properties of nicotine. Some of these controls are needed for any drug that is studied in this paradigm, whereas others are necessitated by the specific traits of nicotine. In the next chapter we will review the research in nicotine self-administration in animals. We will see that as a rule, the requisite controls were not employed and, as a result, the role of nicotine as a reinforcer in this paradigm has not been adequately established.

Chapter 6

THE REINFORCING PROPERTIES OF
NICOTINE IN ANIMALS

This chapter aims to scrutinize the evidence for the proposition that nicotine is reinforcing in animals. The majority of the chapter is dedicated to examining the claim that animals will self-administer pure nicotine, either orally or by intravenous injection.

The last sections of this chapter evaluate whether the classical conditioning paradigms of conditioned taste aversion and conditioned place preference support the claim that nicotine is reinforcing to animals.

1.   ORAL SELF-ADMINISTRATION OF NICOTINE

There is no doubt that animals, under certain conditions, can be forced to self-administer all drugs. Investigators determine such conditions for reasons other than to test whether a given drug has reinforcing properties. Often the motivation is to save time: rather than manually injecting the animal daily with a particular drug, the investigator forces the animals to self-administer the drugs. In such experiments the animals are generally confronted with a no-choice situation. For example, the drug may be dissolved in drinking water, and as this is the only source of water available to the animal, it will drink the solution and thereby self-administer the drug. Of course, such forced self-administration has no bearing on the question of whether or not a given drug is reinforcing. To demonstrate that a drug has reinforcing properties, the animal must have a choice between a drug and a no-drug alternative. For instance, the animal can be confronted with two water bottles – one containing plain water and the other water mixed with nicotine. If the animal prefers to drink the nicotine solution, we may conclude that nicotine is more reinforcing than plain water in this setting.

Only a small minority of studies reported that certain animals, such as the tree shrew[468], prefer drinking nicotine solution to water. The general finding is that rats, mice, and squirrel monkeys normally do not prefer nicotine solutions to water[180,301,530]. Nevertheless, two recent reports claim to have demonstrated a preference for oral nicotine over control solutions in rats. We will discuss them in some detail, not because these experiments prove that nicotine is reinforcing, but because they demonstrate some of the pitfalls of this line of research.

The first report, by Smith and Roberts[613], describes four experiments. The first study aimed to investigate "*whether rats could be induced to consume nicotine orally* (p. 342)" by adding sucrose to nicotine solution. The study showed that adding sucrose indeed induced the rats to consume the nicotine solution. However, the intake of sucrose + nicotine never exceeded that of sucrose taken alone, and in two concentration levels was significantly lower. In other words, the rats preferred their sucrose pure, without nicotine.

The second experiment in this study was designed to see whether rats would perform an operant response for nicotine reward. The rats were housed in operant chambers containing *ad libitum* food and water, as well as a lever and a cup. For one group of rats, pressing the lever would squirt a small amount of a sucrose solution into the cup. For the second group of animals, a lever press would produce the same amount of sucrose solution mixed with nicotine. Thus, rather than having free access to sweet water or sweet water + nicotine, the animals now had to work for their reward. The results showed that the rats that were reinforced with sucrose + nicotine tended to press the lever somewhat more than the rats that received only sucrose, but this difference did not even approach statistical significance (p was 0.27). Furthermore, there is a simple explanation for this small difference. For an unspecified reason, the rats who were to be trained to work for sucrose + nicotine were maintained on the same sweet nicotine solution two weeks prior to the training, and then continued to have free access to this solution between the operant training trials. As a result, these rats must have been highly aroused, which fully accounts for their slight tendency to press the lever more frequently. In any case, the results of this experiment indicate that the animals did *not* press for nicotine. When the sucrose concentration was gradually reduced, the rats receiving sweet water + nicotine reduced their response at exactly the same rate as the rats who were receiving just the sucrose solution, which strongly suggests that they pressed for sucrose, not for nicotine.

In the third experiment in this study[613], the fixed ratio was gradually increased from FR5 to FR20. As the ratio increased (i.e., rats had to press more to obtain a droplet of solution), and specifically between FR7 and FR16, sucrose + nicotine reinforced rats pressed more frequently than rats reinforced with sucrose alone. The authors concluded, on the basis of these findings, that "*sucrose + nicotine solutions are more reinforcing than sucrose solutions alone* (p. 341)." In making this unequivocal statement, which appears in the abstract of the article, Smith and Roberts apparently did not consider the alternative explanations discussed in the previous chapter. Specifically, the increased response rate of the nicotine + sucrose rats could be due to nicotine's augmentation of general activation and, especially in the higher reinforcement schedules, to its enhancement of memory consolidation.

Notably, Smith and Roberts seem to have been aware of the severe limitations of their study. In the discussion section of their article, they added this qualification: "*It must be emphasized that the enhanced responding for the SUC + NIC solution was demonstrated in animals that had been ingesting nicotine for several months. Whether animals with less experience with nicotine would respond to higher FR values is presently unknown* (p. 345)." Moreover, in contrast to the decisive wording in the abstract, their conclusion in the body of the article is carefully stated: "*When a response criterion is enforced, the response maintaining effects of sweetened nicotine solutions are greater than those of comparable sucrose-only solutions* (p. 345)." The difference between "response maintaining" and "reinforcing" is telling. As we showed earlier, nicotine (and other drugs) can maintain response without possessing primary reinforcing properties. Indeed, a subsequent study of oral nicotine preference confirmed that increased response rate in these paradigms is attributable to the general activating effects of nicotine.

In this later study, Glick, Visker, and Maisonneuve[212] used a different procedure than that of Smith and Roberts. They placed rats in operant chambers equipped with *two* levers and *two* cups. The rats were deprived of water for 23 hours per day and then trained to press for plain water for one hour.   Both levers were 'active,' so that pressing on either lever was rewarded with a droplet of water in the cup above that lever.   After the rats had acquired stable levels of lever pressing, nicotine solutions were introduced.   A press on lever A squirted plain water, whereas a press on lever B produced a nicotine solution.   The levers were alternated every session. The concentration of nicotine was doubled once a week.

This two-lever choice situation demonstrated unequivocally that nicotine produces general activation which, in this setting, was expressed in frequency of lever pressing.   The most significant finding in this study was that as nicotine levels were increased, the rate of lever pressing *on both levers* increased in a parallel fashion (from about 100 per hour at a nicotine concentration of 4 µg/ml to 160 per hour at a nicotine concentration of 32 µg/ml).   This finding supports our contention that what Smith and Roberts[613] reported as a reinforcing effect of nicotine was most likely a non-specific stimulant effect.

What about preference for nicotine over plain water?   The investigators reported that 16 of the 20 rats *"reliably preferred bar-pressing to receive nicotine, at 4–32 µg/ml, than to receive water* (p. 427)[212]*."*   However, no significance tests of these differences are reported, and the meaning of "reliably" remains unclear.   The authors do report that four rats (20 percent) never preferred nicotine.   Did all of the other 16 rats prefer nicotine at every concentration level in this range, in all of the sessions?   The data are aggregated in a way that does not disclose this information.   Moreover, a recent report from the same group, using identical methodology, indicates that the finding that 80 percent of the rats preferred nicotine in the Glick, Visker, and Maisonneuve study is in fact quite *unreliable.*   For their second study[211], the researchers selected only rats that demonstrated a preference for nicotine in this paradigm.   In parentheses, they explain that *"not all rats have nicotine preference"* and, specifically, *"approximately 50 percent of the rats screened for this study had nicotine preferences* (p. 275)[211]*."*   Inexplicably, the contradiction between these figures and those reported in the original study goes unnoticed by Glick and his colleagues.   Obviously, if only 50 percent of the rats prefer nicotine in this paradigm, it must relinquish its claim as "*an oral self administration model of nicotine preference in rats* (p. 426)[212,D]."

2.   INTRAVENOUS SELF-ADMINISTRATION

The problems caused by nicotine's bad taste can be circumvented by training animals to self-administer nicotine intravenously. This procedure has been successfully employed for other drugs. With most psychoactive drugs, however, it produces much stronger evidence of reinforcement than it does with nicotine. Specifically, known psychoactive drugs, including opiates[60,408,451,674,721] and cocaine[60] [716]not only maintain lever pressing for self-administration, but are also sufficiently reinforcing to initiate such behavior. In contrast, under normal conditions, animals do not initiate nicotine self-administration, either orally or intravenously. Only a few reports claim otherwise, and these are all problematic. In one report[122], for example, rats received multiple nicotine injections prior to intravenous nicotine self-administration, and nicotine increased response rates for both the 'active' (delivering nicotine) and the 'inactive' lever; therefore, as discussed earlier, this result is attributable to general behavior activation. A more recent study[667] also failed to employ adequate control for the activating effects of nicotine, and even so, the majority of its results were not statistically significant.

In other experiments reporting marginal preference for nicotine self-administration[e.g.,601,603,605], animals received a "priming injection" of nicotine prior to each session. Such "priming" can obviously affect performance in later trials, a possibility that can be easily examined, for example, by including a control group that would receive the priming

---

[D] We should note that even if a reliable majority of rats in Glick, Visker, and Maisonneuve's study[212] did press the lever that squirted nicotine more often than the one that squirted water, their conclusion that nicotine is therefore reinforcing would still be problematic. First, the researchers only measured how often the rats pressed and not their actual consumption of fluids; therefore, there is no evidence that the rats actually *drank* more nicotine solution than water. Second, if nicotine had been reinforcing, there should have been a learning curve showing a gradual increase in lever pressing for nicotine, relative to water, during every 1-hour session and between sessions for each nicotine concentration level. The authors did not present any data to show that such learning occurred.

injections but would later self-administer only saline. No such group was included, however. In another recent study, which purportedly demonstrated that nicotine can initiate self- administration[390], animals were food-restricted, some were nicotine-"primed," and no controls for general activation were used.

The fact that, unlike known addictive drugs, nicotine is not unconditionally self-administered by animals argues strongly against it being a potent reinforcer. But even the claim that nicotine will maintain self-administration is very weakly substantiated. We found that most studies that have made this claim contained fundamental methodological flaws, particularly a surprising lack of controls for the non-reinforcing effects of nicotine discussed in the previous chapter. With the exception of a handful of studies, to be discussed in detail later, there was little attempt to rule out such alternative explanations. The fact that animals can be made to self-administer nicotine in the same paradigm where they also self-administer heroin, cocaine, and other known reinforcing drugs, seems to be taken as evidence that nicotine must be as reinforcing as heroin or cocaine. The flaw in this argument is obvious. The syllogism: "Animals self-administer all reinforcing drugs; Animals self-administer nicotine; Hence nicotine is a reinforcing drug" is as false as the syllogism: "People eat all animals; People eat coleslaw; Hence coleslaw is an animal."

2.1   The Early Studies (until 1989)

Even when animals were first trained to press a lever for another reinforcer such as food and then were switched to nicotine injections, early studies often failed to demonstrate nicotine self-administration[21,122,234,729]. When self-administration occurred[21,149,253,366,612,616,729], it was often marginal, not dose-related, or demonstrated only in food-deprived animals (a limitation we will discuss later in this chapter). Several studies[e.g.,21,136,214,219,220,612,623] used very few subjects and presented almost no statistics. Often the animals had participated in earlier studies where they had been trained to self-administer food, or known reinforcing drugs such as cocaine. Some of the studies reporting success and quoted by the Surgeon General are available only in abstract form and thus do not permit scrutiny of the methods[e.g.,215,504].

A 1988 review[217] concluded: *"The series of studies reviewed show that nicotine by itself can serve as an effective reinforcer for humans and experimental animals, but it does so under a more limited range of conditions than do other reinforcers such as IV cocaine injection or food presentation."* It is precisely this "limited range of conditions" that should have motivated every experimenter to employ a maximum of controls. "A limited range of conditions" means that the reliability of animal models for intravenous self-administration of nicotine is poor, and therefore, alternative explanations should be given most serious consideration.

Referring to these early self-administration studies, Corrigall and Coen[115] wrote: *"While these studies have suggested that nicotine might serve as a reinforcer in rodents, they have not provided convincing evidence."* We concur. Indeed, what was considered the most convincing evidence by the Surgeon General and most investigators during the 1980s were not rodent studies, but primarily primate studies. The most influential of them was a 1981 article in *Science*, authored by Goldberg, Spealman and Goldberg. According to the Surgeon General, *"Goldberg, Spealman, and Goldberg showed conclusively that nicotine itself could function as an efficacious positive reinforcer for animals, although the range of conditions under which it was effective was somewhat more limited than for drugs such as cocaine and amphetamine* (p. 181)[665]*."* Because of its influence, and especially its central place in the Surgeon General's report, this study merits detailed analysis.

The total sample in this "conclusive" study[220] consisted of four squirrel monkeys. The animals sat in chairs in a sound-attenuated chamber and could operate a single response lever. Pressing the lever produced a brief light stimulus that was occasionally associated with an intravenous injection of nicotine. This second-order reinforcement schedule produced a gradual increase in rate of responding. Furthermore, substituting nicotine with saline injections or blocking nicotine receptors with mecamylamine resulted in a marked reduction in the rate of lever pressing.

Disregarding the small sample, these results appear convincing at first glance. However, a first glance is often deceptive. The authors never considered, at least not in writing, two well-established facts that constitute obvious alternative explanations for their findings. First of all, as discussed at length earlier, nicotine induces general activation in animals[16,35,68,98,99,102,117,118,153,248,260,322,361,433,438,441,457,519,521,544,571,574,579,604,633,695].

As lever pressing was the only available activity for the monkeys, nicotine would be expected to increase lever pressing. When saline was substituted for the nicotine, the activation level, and consequently the rate of lever pressing, would be expected to drop. Furthermore, as mecamylamine blocks the stimulant effects of nicotine[99,102], it would be expected to block the increase in lever pressing induced by the general activating property of nicotine.

Moreover, of the four monkeys, only one was naive; the other three had been trained to press the lever for cocaine. No rationale is given for the cocaine pre-training – presumably, the authors could not otherwise get this threesome to press for nicotine reward. The cocaine-trained monkeys were submitted to a saline extinction schedule. Such extinction, however, is limited, and in this case it clearly did not cause the monkeys to forget having received cocaine for lever pressing. This is evident from the fact that *"in the cocaine-trained monkeys, responding was established under a second-order schedule of intravenous nicotine without preliminary training* (p. 573)." Cocaine is a powerful reinforcer. It is powerful enough to facilitate second-order conditioning as well as to transfer secondary reinforcing properties, by classical conditioning, to the lever the animals had been pressing. As intravenous nicotine injection is a salient cue in animals[90,575,602], it could become associated with the secondary reinforcing properties of the lever that was previously conditioned to the reinforcing effects of cocaine and thereby enhance responding as a secondary reinforcer. In addition to these two crucial alternative mechanisms, there is another possibility that Goldberg, Spealman and Goldberg[220] did not entertain: rats in a stimulus-free environment are willing to work for the light stimulus itself. The fact that light is reinforcing for rats was recognized and studied in the operant chamber over two decades ago[e.g.,254,440,714] but seems to have been forgotten by modern researchers. While there is no direct evidence that monkeys will acquire level pressing with a light reward, it is certainly a possibility that must be considered in interpreting the results of this study.

The authors of this study, then, demonstrated a disregard of alternative explanations of their findings. Unfortunately, as we note throughout this book, this type of confirmatory bias is all too common in research on nicotine addiction. In addition, the design of the study was seriously flawed. There were five manipulations in all (nicotine + mecamylamine, nicotine + no light, saline, saline + no light, and resumption of nicotine), but the design was not fully crossed: Saline was substituted for nicotine only in the three cocaine-trained monkeys; mecamylamine was administered only to two of the four monkeys, and the same was the case for omitting the light stimulus. Only one monkey received all five manipulations, and the lone nicotine-trained monkey received only two manipulations. In addition, the authors did not provide any statistical analysis of the data, or even tables of results, so we are left to judge the results by eyeballing the figures. In the same vein, there are no standard definitions for a "reduction" or an "increase" in the rate of pressing. To illustrate, one monkey (S-156) increased its pressing rate by 0.7 responses per second during the four baseline sessions. When the light stimulus was omitted, another monkey (S-464) is said to have reduced its pressing rate, but this supposed reduction is only by 0.4 responses per second. Thus, in one case, a difference of 0.4 responses per second is considered a meaningful reduction, while in another case, an increase of 0.7 responses per second is dismissed as baseline variability.

The order and length of the manipulations in Goldberg, Spealman and Goldberg's[220] study is neither fixed nor counterbalanced. In fact, there is only one manipulation that two monkeys (S-200 and S-464) share in the same order: The light stimulus is omitted after four baseline sessions and reinstated afterwards. Out of a total of 18 manipulations in this study, three consisted of two sessions, five of four sessions, one of five sessions, three of six sessions, one of seven sessions, two of nine sessions, two of ten sessions and one of eleven sessions. The length of the manipulations seems to have been determined *ad hoc* by whether the results were in the predicted direction. In the above example of omitting the light stimulus, one monkey was run for seven sessions and the other for eleven sessions before the light stimulus was reinstated. The experimenters must have waited until each monkey was at a visible low point, and then stopped (thus eliminating the risk that the response rate would increase again). The same pattern was repeated when the light was reinstated. The first monkey returned to baseline levels after five sessions, at which point observations were stopped (thereby avoiding the risk of a later reduction in the rate of pressing). In contrast, thesecond animal was observed with patience for eleven sessions, until it finally returned to its baseline levels[E].

[E] To verify that the implied relationship between the number of sessions and the animal's cooperation with the experimental hypotheses is not merely an unfair prejudice, we conducted

This is the study, then, that provided a "conclusive demonstration," at least for the Surgeon General, that nicotine can function as an efficacious positive reinforcer[665]. This conclusive demonstration relied on a total of four monkeys, of which only two were subjected to the critical manipulations, with no control for general activation, no standardization of procedure, no statistical tests of the results or even numerical summaries of the data and no consideration of alternative explanations of the findings. But then again, relative to other evidence the Surgeon General had at his disposal for his 1988 report, this study[220] may well have been the best case for self-administration of nicotine by animals.

2.2   Limitations of Recent Studies (1989-1999)

A year following the Surgeon General's report, a new method of nicotine self-administration in the rat was described by Corrigall and Coen[115]. According to the authors, the new method resulted in relatively high, stable, and dose-dependent rates of responding, without the use of concurrent additional reinforcement or nicotine pretreatment. Corrigall and Coen's method was replicated many times by their group and several others[e.g., 31,94,116,117,118,119,120,147,148,471,489,490,595,651,689]. Nevertheless, the procedure has major drawbacks, which severely limit the conclusions that can be drawn from it.

2.2.1   Food Deprivation

According to Corrigall and Coen's method, rats are food deprived for 36 hours, and then trained to press a lever for food pellets on a continuous reinforcement schedule (FR1 – a food pellet is delivered on each press). Once trained, animals are fed their daily nutrient requirement of standard lab chow as a single meal (20g). Following training, an intravenous catheter is

---

the following analysis. For each manipulation, we computed a 'favorable change index,' using the difference in pressing rates (in the predicted direction) between the last session of the prior condition and the second session of the present manipulation. We then correlated this index with the number of sessions the researchers allowed for this manipulation. The Spearman rank correlation was -0.72 ($p < 0.05$), so that smaller changes in the expected direction were significantly related to a larger number of sessions. Of course, a correlation does not imply causation.

implanted in the rats and they are put in an operant chamber for one hour each day. They have access to the same lever they had learned to press under previous training conditions, but rather than receiving a food pellet as a reinforcement, they receive an injection of nicotine solution. The other training conditions are also maintained. Specifically, the animals continue to be fed 20g of food following the session, which is about *half* of what they would eat if they had free access to food[148]. They cannot eat again until after the next session, at least 20 hours later. Thus, as Corrigall and Coen[115] acknowledged, the rats are not only food deprived throughout the study, but are particularly hungry during the nicotine self-administration sessions.

Food deprivation in rats is a facilitating condition for nicotine self-administration, as shown earlier by others[e.g.,149,366,609]. A more recent demonstration was provided by Watkins et al.[689]. These authors used basically the same method as Corrigall and Coen[115] for training the animals, but fed their animals *ad libitum* when pressing for nicotine. This had a dramatic effect on self-administration: in one of their experiments, only 6 out of 17 rats self-administered nicotine. When the animals were returned to the restrictive feeding schedule, 14 of 17 self-administered nicotine. Thus, Watkins et al.[689] unintentionally performed a much-needed control experiment. Their findings suggest that the critical factor in Corrigall and Coen's[115] procedure is hunger, rather than nicotine. Animals that were trained to press a lever for food will continue to do so whenever they are hungry. This is not surprising, as in Corrigall and Coen's procedure, animals do not go through an extinction period before they are switched to nicotine. As Donny et al.[148] demonstrated, prior operant conditioning with food reinforcement can sustain bar pressing in hungry animals in the absence of nicotine or food for at least nine days. This finding suggests that the reinforcing properties of food for hungry animals may be transferred, by classical conditioning, to the lever. The secondary reinforcing properties of the lever can later be conditioned to any recognizable stimulus property of nicotine and make its injection reinforcing.

This hypothesis is supported by the observations of Shaham and his co-authors[595] that acutely food-deprived rats, trained to self-administer nicotine and then subsequently extinguished, display not only nicotine-seeking, but also food-seeking behavior, following a priming injection of nicotine. Together, these studies suggest that self-administration of nicotine in Corrigall and Coen's[115] paradigm may be due to secondary reinforcing properties acquired by classical conditioning to food. However, as we shall show in the next sections, it is more likely that nicotine in this paradigm either did not enhance lever-pressing at all, or did so by facilitating ongoing behavior of the animals rather than acting as a reinforcer.

The possibility that hunger is the crucial factor that maintains nicotine self-administration in Corrigall and Coen's paradigm is also consistent with the well-known anorectic properties of nicotine in rats[e.g.,588,734]. This anorectic effect could well be sufficiently reinforcing to sustain responding, even if nicotine would have no reinforcing properties in any other condition. Through this mechanism nicotine acts as a negative reinforcer, not a positive one, that is, the animals self-administer nicotine in order to reduce their hunger.

2.2.2   Elimination of Uncooperative Subjects

The original study that made Corrigall and Coen's procedure popular[115] did not control for the effects of weight and food restriction on nicotine self-administration. The first attempt to validate Corrigall and Coen's model by submitting it to systematic, critical, and well-controlled experimentation was undertaken by Donny and his colleagues nine years later[148]. Because the findings of this study were interpreted by the authors as validating Corrigall and Coen's paradigm, it is important to examine it closely.

Donny and his colleagues conducted three separate studies, designed to examine the effects of nicotine dose, feeding schedule and drug contingency on lever pressing (and consequent nicotine infusion) in Corrigall and Coen's[115] procedure. In the first study, they showed that rats trained according to this procedure self-administered nicotine at doses of 0.03 and 0.06 mg/kg per infusion. Nicotine self-administration was defined as a statistically significant difference between the frequency of pressing on the active as compared to the inactive lever. However, these significant differences were obtained on a biased sub-sample of the rats: animals that did not achieve stable nicotine self-administration were excluded from analysis. In the 0.06 mg/kg dose, one third of the rats were excluded from the reported results; for the 0.03 mg/kg dose, 40 percent of the rats were excluded. The authors stated that *"the same pattern of results was found when all animals were included in the analyses, indicating that the results are not a function of an arbitrary acquisition criterion* (p. 85)[148]." However, this "pattern" is not presented, and we seriously doubt that the statistical analyses would have produced the same results; otherwise, there would have been no need to exclude the uncooperative subjects.

The peculiar practice of excluding animals that do not meet the desirable performance criteria from data analysis and from the reported results seems to be the rule in this paradigm[e.g.,31,116,117,118,147,595,603,689]. Whether this was also done by other groups is often not clear from the methods[e.g.,94,119,120,471]. Discarding animals from analyses may be valid for some questions, but it can radically distort reality when as many as half of the animals are excluded for failing to acquire nicotine self-administration[e.g.,603]. Exclusion of uncooperative animals is clearly not appropriate when the research question is whether or not rats self-administer nicotine. By discarding animals that do not perform in the way that the investigator wishes, almost any desirable result can be obtained. As noted earlier, excluding animals that do not self-administer nicotine (about half of the population) and then proceeding to draw general conclusions appears to be an accepted norm in oral self-administration studies as well[e.g.,211].

In their second experiment, Donny and his co-authors[148] examined the effect of food and weight restriction on lever pressing and the resultant amount of self-administered nicotine. The results confirmed that the practice of restricting the animals' diet and depriving them of food for more than 20 hours prior to each session are crucial factors in this paradigm. Animals that had unlimited access to food during the nicotine sessions pressed the lever about 3 times less, and self-administered about one-third nicotine, compared to the animals that were food-deprived and weight-restricted. This overwhelming effect did not deter the authors from concluding that "*SA is not dependent on deprivation and/or weight restriction,*" as "*rats in all feeding conditions demonstrated clear evidence of nicotine self-administration* (p. 88)." Even the second part of this statement, however, is invalid for the reason noted above for the first experiment: The statistically significant effect of active vs. inactive lever pressing for the non-deprived group was achieved after 40 percent of the rats that failed to meet self-administration criteria were excluded from analysis.

2.2.3   Lack of Saline Control Groups

There is another serious flaw in the two studies described above, and for that matter, in all but one of the studies that used Corrigall and Coen's procedure: None of these experiments included a saline control group. A saline control group, treated identically to the nicotine self-administering experimental group, is essential for concluding that nicotine has reinforcing effects in food-deprived animals. Instead of saline control conditions, Donny et al.[148], like other researchers using Corrigall and Coen's procedure, considered responding on the inactive lever as their control. Pressing on this inactive lever, however, never produces reinforcement for the animal in this procedure – neither when it is trained with food reward, nor in later stages. Therefore, animals in this procedure learn perfectly well that pressing this lever has no consequences, and demonstrate this knowledge by rarely touching it. Indeed, we know so little about what goes on in a rat's brain that we cannot even be certain that rats recognize an inactive lever as a lever! As far as we can tell, this control is worthless both for measuring non-specific activation and most certainly for assessing extinction of pressing for food reward. This was demonstrated directly by Bardo and his coworkers[31]. They used the same procedure as Donny and his co-authors but also had a control group pressing for saline injections. During the first 5 days of training in an FR1 schedule, there was no observable difference between the saline and the nicotine reinforced group. Thus, whatever pressing occurred during this phase of self-administration is entirely attributable to lack of extinction of pressing for food-reward, rather to any effect of nicotine.

That animals had not in fact undergone extinction is also evident from the third experiment of Donny et al.[148] (see also Shaham et al.[595]), where saline controls pressed about 25 times during the first session, and complete extinction had not been achieved during the 9 days of the study. In our opinion, the omission of saline control groups, combined with the practice of excluding one-third to one-half of the animals that do not acquire nicotine self-administration, invalidates Donny et al's first two experiments, as well as most other studies in the same paradigm[e.g.,116,117,118,147,595,603,689].

2.2.4   Limited Evidence for Drug Contingency Effects

The third experiment in Donny et al. was designed to examine the effects of drug contingency on lever pressing for nicotine. Each rat that was run in the usual procedure had two yoked controls. Every time it pressed a lever, the first yoked subject received a nicotine infusion identical to the self-administered one, and the second yoked animal received an infusion of saline solution. For the yoked controls, then, infusions were not contingent on lever pressing. This method is useful for separating the general effects of nicotine discussed above, particularly general activation, from its rewarding properties. Specifically, a difference between the nicotine self-administering group and the yoked nicotine group would indicate that lever pressing could not be accounted for by general activation, as the latter should be the same in these two groups. Indeed, the self-administering group in this experiment pressed the lever significantly more than the two yoked control groups, which did not differ between them and in which responses gradually declined over the nine days of the study.

Although these results are potentially important, this single experiment does not provide sufficient grounds for concluding that nicotine is self-administered in this paradigm for its rewarding properties. A replication is always a requirement in science, but it is especially needed in this case not only because of the numerous negative results reviewed above, but also because of three anomalies in this particular experiment. First, there was no evidence in this experiment of the general activation effects of nicotine, which should have been expressed in more lever pressing overall in the yoked nicotine group as compared to the yoked saline group, especially during the later phases of the study. This lack of general activation effect is peculiar in light of studies cited above[e.g.,122,667], in which nicotine-administering animals showed considerable elevations in both active and inactive lever pressing. Second, the self-administering rats pressed twice as many times as the other two groups *in the very first session*. As lever pressing in the first session is mostly determined by prior conditioning to food reward, this finding is peculiar and suggests that the results of this experiment reflect initial differences between the three groups. Third, the contingency group in this experiment, from which no animals were discarded, pressed nearly twice as many times as contingency groups in the two earlier experiments, where up to 40 percent of the animals were discarded for not meeting the criterion. This observation is consistent with the possibility that the contingency group in this particular experiment was anomalous, and its higher pressing rate reflects baseline differences rather than the reinforcing effects of nicotine.

2.2.5   Confounding Reinforcement with Activation

In several studies that employed Corrigall and Coen's procedure[e.g.,31,147,148,651], rats were submitted to fixed ratio (non-continuous) schedules of reinforcement. These schedules (FR2 and FR5) generally led to an increase in responding, which was taken as evidence for the reinforcing properties of nicotine. However, this conclusion is dubious, especially in view of a recent study by Bardo and coworkers[31]. As in similar studies, rats were allowed a number of days (five, in this case) on an FR1 schedule before switching to higher ratio schedules. Rather than increased responding over these five days, which would indicate learning, rats showed a reduction in responses until day 5. More importantly, response rates were not noticeably different from the response rates for saline during these five days. Thus, by these two criteria, when animals were on the FR1 schedule, nicotine did *not* act as a reinforcer. However, when animals were switched for two days to an FR2 and for 5 days to an FR5 schedule, lever-pressing rate increased two-fold and five-fold, respectively. Though the authors did not comment on this pattern, we find it quite puzzling: How could nicotine be reinforcing in FR2 and FR5 schedules, but not in the continuous reinforcement (FR1) schedule?

We propose that the answer is to be found in another experiment by the same group of investigators[153]. This study demonstrated that a pharmacologically similar dose of nicotine (0.3–1.0 mg/kg) as self-administered in the previous study (about 0.6 mg per session) will produce a depression of locomotion at the first daily session, but enhanced locomotion by Day 8. In other words, rats self-administering nicotine will become increasingly activated (and hence press more) following daily exposures to nicotine, in a timeframe that corresponds to shifting the animals to FR2 and FR5 schedules in the first study. With the exception of the study described above by Donny and his co-workers[148], this crucial confound has not been controlled for by any of the studies using Corrigall and Coen's procedure.

2.3   Other Recent Animal Self-Administration Studies

As stated earlier, the study by Donny and his co-workers.[148] seems to have been the only attempt to validate Corrigall and Coen's model. The vast majority of the experiments performed after 1989 were not designed to test whether animals self-administer nicotine because of its reinforcing properties. Instead, they were designed to test further manipulations on what were *assumed* to be reinforcing properties of nicotine in rats[e.g.,94,471,490], monkeys[562,679], and mice[406]. Generally, investigators in this field seem to believe that the issue has been settled, despite the lack of studies that convincingly reject any of the multiple alternative explanations of the data.

A recent study with mice employed a different procedure from that of Corrigall and Coen's. Stolerman et al.[636] trained water-deprived mice to press a lever for water, and then switched them to intravenous nicotine. Animals self-administered first a higher dose of nicotine, than a lower dose, and finally saline, each for six daily sessions. The authors observed a significant increase in responses over the six days of the higher dose, a significant decrease over the six days of the lower dose, and no change over the six days that the animals received saline.

Unfortunately, this design also suffers from methodological problems. The order of the nicotine dose was not counter-balanced, so it was completely confounded with the time factor. Thus, any changes with the nicotine dose may be attributable to the effects of time on memory, activation or suppression of motor responses, and most importantly, on extinction. Furthermore, only the high dose of nicotine, which was administered immediately following training with water reward, was significantly different from saline, and even this effect was obtained only by omitting the first three days of each dose from the analysis. In fact, saline maintained responding for six days, without any decline in response rate, at levels that were indistinguishable from the lower nicotine dose. Thus, the results of this study can be fully accounted for by the effects of nicotine on activation together with the secondary reinforcing properties that nicotine has acquired from the water reward.

Two other studies with mice demonstrated a more careful approach to experimental design and control[406,515]. These investigators had mice nose-poke for injections. The animals were placed in a confining experimental chamber with their tails outside. The tail was prepared with an intravenous catheter and fixed to the floor with adhesive tape. The only behavior the animals could perform was poking their nose through an opening in the wall. Half of the animals received an injection of nicotine or saline contingent upon this "nose-poke," while the other half served as passive yoked controls, receiving the injection whenever their active partner nose poked. As mentioned above, this is an excellent way to control for general activation.

In both studies, the "contingent" animals poked significantly more than the yoked controls on two doses of nicotine. These studies demonstrate, therefore, that nicotine seems to have reinforcing properties in immobilized mice. Clearly, these results are somewhat limited in scope. Immobilizing mice is a manipulation that increases stress[e.g.,93,639,668], and more studies will have to be conducted to see whether stress is a necessary condition for these effects to occur. Moreover, nose-poking in mice is apparently a spontaneous (not learned) behavior and baseline or control levels of some groups in the same study (e.g., for cocaine and epibatidine) were nearly as high as the poking rates induced by nicotine[515]. Also, the observation that the reinforcing effects of nicotine did not require learning is puzzling, as is the absence of any general activating effects. However, in contrast to the vast majority of nicotine self-administration studies, these studies are carefully designed and executed. To date, these seem to be the only well-controlled studies in which animals that were neither food deprived nor trained on other reinforcements initiated self-administration of nicotine.

3. DEMONSTRATING REINFORCING PROPERTIES OF DRUGS USING CLASSICAL CONDITIONING

As discussed in the previous chapter, self-administration is not sufficient evidence for the reinforcing properties of a drug. One reason for that is the fact that drugs can become secondary reinforcers by classical conditioning to primary reinforcers such as food. However, classical conditioning itself can also be exploited to elucidate the reinforcing properties of drugs. Like Skinner, in his experiments with instrumental conditioning, Pavlov knew the (primary) reinforcing properties of the stimuli he used: meat powder is rewarding to dogs, pain is aversive. Therefore, as in the case of instrumental conditioning, the logic of the classical conditioning experiments can be reversed. If the reinforcing properties of a given drug (positive, negative, or none at all) are unknown, the drug can be paired with neutral stimuli. Subsequently, it can be inferred from the behavior of the experimental subjects, whether those neutral stimuli become secondary positive or negative reinforcers. Will the subjects *approach* those formerly neutral stimuli following conditioning, or will they *avoid* them?

Naturally, the classical conditioning paradigm is prone to the same problems as the self-administration paradigm. If many drug injections are needed to produce conditioning, physical dependence may confound the results. But if only few, or better, only one drug injection has to be paired with a neutral stimulus to produce conditioning, then the researcher can safely conclude that the drug in question is a primary positive reinforcer. Fortunately, there are two classical conditioning paradigms that meet this requirement: **conditioned taste aversion** and **conditioned place preference**. These names are misleading: Although the first paradigm is called 'taste aversion' and the second 'place preference,' both paradigms can be used to demonstrate both aversions and preferences.

3.1 Conditioned Taste Aversion

John Garcia's well-known experiments on the phenomenon of conditioned taste aversion (CTA) constitute one of the most impressive research programs in the area of animal and human learning. In his first experiment[199], rats were exposed to food with a novel flavor. After the rats ate, half of them received an injection of a poison that made them sick and the other half received an injection of saline. Animals that were not made sick ate the food with the novel taste several days later. Animals that had been sick, though they have by now recovered, did not eat the food. In subsequent experiments, Garcia and his coworkers showed that the aversion the rats have developed was specific to the flavor, and that every agent that makes animals sick will produce CTA[200]. Conversely, when a novel taste is paired with reward, the result is conditioned taste *preference*.

Interestingly, when psychoactive drugs are paired with a novel taste in animals, they usually produce conditioned taste aversion, rather than preference. Systemically administered amphetamine[372,597], cocaine[173,615], alcohol[125], the active ingredient of hashish (delta-THC)[474], and morphine[372,596] have all been demonstrated to produce CTA in rats. In fact, we are not certain that there exists a single psychoactive drug that is self-administered by humans and does *not* produce CTA in animals. It is therefore not surprising that nicotine was also found to produce conditioned taste aversion[e.g.,469].

The CTA paradigm, therefore, appears to be singularly unsuitable for discriminating rewarding from non-rewarding drugs – according to this paradigm, none of the psychoactive drugs is rewarding. This observation raises an important theoretical question. In view of the fact that all of the chemicals mentioned above are self-administered by humans and some of them, at least, must have rewarding properties, why are they also aversive?

There is no answer to this question that is accepted by all workers in the field, various explanations for this finding have been raised[e.g., 235]. The most parsimonious explanation is based on the fact that psychoactive drugs are administered systemically. As these drugs interfere with normal neural transmission in the brain, it is more than likely that the neurotransmitters affected by the drug are involved in many different brain systems that are responsible for a multitude of behaviors[706]. Some of these brain systems normally produce aversive effects, and others rewarding effects. This idea is supported by observations[e.g.,596,597] that psychoactive drugs can produce CTA and conditioned place preference (CPP) *simultaneously* in the same animal.

3.2   Conditioned Place Preference

Conditioned place preference (CPP) is another classical conditioning paradigm that can be used to demonstrate reinforcing properties of substances. In its simplest form, the animal is first exposed to a cage with two distinctly different chambers. After it is established that the animal has no preference for either chamber, meaning that it will spend an equal amount of time in each one, the animal is injected with a drug while it is in one of the chambers. A few days later, when the effects of the drug have worn off, the animal is tested again. If it now shows a preference for the chamber in which it was injected, the conclusion is that the drug had positive reinforcing properties. If the animal shows an aversion towards that chamber by spending more time in the other one, or has no preference for either chamber, the drug had apparently no rewarding properties.

CPP in rats following systemic injections of amphetamine[e.g.,625], [32,661]cocaine[e.g.,70], and morphine[e.g.,436] has been reliably demonstrated. This is not the case for alcohol, which produces place preference in mice[e.g.,126] and place aversion in rats[125], even when the drug is self-administered.

Evidence for nicotine-induced CPP is much weaker. Some experiments showed no effect of acute systemic nicotine on place preference[97,473]. Others found place aversion[328]. Some groups found both place preference and place aversion[78,194,195,286,526], depending on various methodological parameters. Only one group of investigators[3,82] observed CPP without aversion, but an attempted replication by others using the same dose[604] did not succeed in reproducing these results. There is therefore no clear or consistent evidence that nicotine produces CPP.

4. CONCLUSIONS

Self-administration studies in animals have not established the role of nicotine as a positive primary reinforcer. The great majority of these studies suffer from severe methodological flaws, which jeopardize both their internal and their external validity. The internal validity of these studies, that is, the extent to which the results could be interpreted as reflecting nicotine self-administration, was compromised by (1) a lack of appropriate comparison groups, particularly saline and yoked controls; (2) partial presentation of results and absence of statistical tests; (3) lack of standardization and *ad hoc* methodological decisions. The external validity of these studies, that is, the extent to which their results can be attributable to the reinforcing properties of nicotine, is limited due to (1) lack of control for general activation, anorectic properties and other systemic effects of nicotine; (2) insufficient consideration of secondary reinforcement processes; (3) using food-deprived or confined animals; and (4) exclusion of subjects that do not conform to the investigators' preferred behavior.

The classical conditioning paradigms corroborate the results obtained with the self-administration studies. Most psychoactive drugs, including nicotine, produce conditioned taste aversion upon acute administration. This procedure, therefore, cannot be used to determine the reinforcing properties of drugs. The conditioned place preference paradigm does seem to detect reinforcing drugs, and in marked contrast to morphine and cocaine, nicotine does not reliably produce CPP. The absence of convincing nicotine-produced place preference, especially in view of the many attempts to elicit it, is inconsistent with the hypothesis that nicotine is reinforcing to animals. We conclude that research does not support the contention that nicotine possesses primary reinforcing properties in animals.

Finally, a central issue in this line of research is the extent to which it is relevant to human tobacco smoking. Even if nicotine were reinforcing in some animals – it is clearly not reinforcing in those animals that were discarded in many studies[e.g.,116,117,118,147,211,595,603,689] – it could still have no role in human smoking.

Indeed, we contend that the conditions under which nicotine self-administration has been obtained in animals are irrelevant to human smoking behavior. A primary example is the fact that in contrast to rats, people like to smoke after a meal, when they are satiated rather than hungry[256,315,318]. Thus, the relevance of rat self-administration studies to humans, even if we put all our other reservations aside, is highly questionable. We shall return to this argument when we discuss the research on the role of nicotine in human tobacco smoking.

Chapter 7

NICOTINE AND INTRACRANIAL SELF-STIMULATION (ICSS)

Self-administration is the principal paradigm used to assess the reinforcing properties of drugs, including nicotine. However, another paradigm, called "intracranial electrical self-stimulation" (ICSS), has also been used for the same purpose. As we aim to show in this chapter, the validity of ICSS for assessing the rewarding properties of drugs is highly questionable. Nevertheless, as nicotine's effects on ICSS have been cited as evidence for its purported reinforcing properties[e.g.,17,37,100,272,299,300,306,732], it is important to explore this paradigm and its implications for the issue of nicotine addiction.

1.   THE ORIGINS OF THE ICSS PARADIGM

Electrical self-stimulation was accidentally discovered in 1954 by Olds and Milner[460]. They observed that rats learned to return to that part of the cage where they had received direct electrical stimulation of the septal area of the brain. This conditioned place preference (see Chapter 6) suggested that the stimulation was rewarding. Olds and Milner subsequently corroborated this hypothesis by training rats to press a lever to electrically self-stimulate locations in their own brains.

Olds and his co-workers soon observed that the extent to which rats were willing to self-stimulate depended primarily on the anatomical area in which the electrode was placed. Rats would press the lever frantically (sometimes up to a hundred times a minute) when the electrode stimulated locations that were involved in rewarding normal behaviors, such as sex, feeding, and drinking. When the electrodes were located in other areas, such as the cerebral cortex, rats did not learn to self-stimulate. Still other electrode locations caused the rats to press the lever in order to stop electrical stimulation. Olds named these locations "reward," "neutral," and "punishment" areas, respectively.

Olds and Milner[460] proposed that ICSS was not essentially different from behavior modification caused by natural rewards. They hypothesized that electrical brain stimulation activated pathways in the brain that are normally activated by natural reinforcers such as food, water, and sexual gratification and, therefore, evoked similar subjective rewards. The main difference between electrical and natural reinforcers, according to Olds and Milner, was in the elimination of the middleman. They believed that electrical stimulation, like natural reinforcers, activated the neural substrate of the reward system, but circumvented the peripheral and central pathways. As we shall see, later research demonstrated that these conclusions were oversimplified.

1.1   The "Pure Incentive" Theory of Self-Stimulation

One of the dominant theoretical accounts of ICSS was proposed by Olds and Olds[461] and Stein[629]. This approach, referred to as the "pure incentive schema[198]," assumed *that the consequences of a behavior pattern, that is, the reward it produces, are responsible for potentiating repetition of behavior. Reward, in other words, operates through a positive feedback amplifier* (p. 181)."

This account of ICSS deviated from the theories of motivation that had dominated experimental psychology for decades in that it disregarded the notion of **drive**. Previous 'homeostatic' theories, to which we will return later, assumed that behavior was potentiated by a 'drive' that generally resulted from a physiological 'need.' The need for food, after deprivation, produced a drive that caused behavior such as foraging and feeding.

'Reward,' in these theories, directed behavior and increased its probability and frequency, but did not produce it. Olds and Olds[461] and Stein[629], in contrast, postulated that ICSS created an 'incentive,' which not only directed behavior but also energized it.

2. THE USE OF ICSS FOR SCREENING PSYCHOACTIVE DRUGS

The idea that ICSS could be a useful paradigm for demonstrating the rewarding properties of psychoactive drugs was introduced in the 1950s. The "pure incentive" theory generated a straightforward hypothesis pertaining to the effects that rewarding drugs should have on ICSS. This hypothesis rested on the three assumptions. First, all neurons in the brain, including those activated by electrical self-stimulation, communicate with each other by releasing neurotransmitters. Second, the neurotransmitters that are released when neurons are stimulated by ICSS in the 'reward areas' are transmitters of 'reward[629].' Until recently, as we will discuss at the end of this chapter, dopamine was believed to be the primary transmitter of reward. Third, psychoactive drugs, particularly those that are habitually self-administered by humans, activate these brain systems of reward and cause the release of, or mimic the action of, the neurotransmitter normally released in these systems. As animals work harder when the reward they receive is greater, injection of a rewarding psychoactive drug should increase rates of self-stimulation. In using ICSS as a screening device, this logic is reversed: if a drug increases self-stimulation, it must be reinforcing to the animal.

Driven by this logic, numerous studies in the past five decades have examined the effects of drugs, including nicotine, on ICSS. Below, we summarize the results of these studies, beginning with morphine and continuing with nicotine. We then proceed to question the adequacy of the ICSS paradigm for exploring the reinforcing properties of drugs and, specifically, of nicotine.

2.1   The Effects of Morphine and Nicotine on ICSS

In summarizing the effects of morphine on ICSS, we restricted ourselves to studies that used medial forebrain bundle (MFB) electrode placements, as the effects of morphine in other locations vary[e.g.,113]. We should also note that even though we will be discussing only the results of morphine, other opiates, notably heroin, have similar effects on ICSS.

The effects of intra-peritoneally administered morphine at doses up to about 5 mg/kg on ICSS are inconsistent. Increases[e.g.,83,213,567,671], decreases[e.g., 387,463,568,573] and no changes in self-stimulation rates[e.g.,568,573,690,693] have been reported.

The effects of higher doses of morphine are more consistent. At doses higher than 5 mg/kg, morphine produces a biphasic effect, first depressing self-stimulation and, about two hours later, increasing it to rates significantly higher than baseline for up to four hours and more[e.g.,6,72,112,252,387,388,462]. With chronic treatment, the depressant effect of morphine undergoes tolerance[e.g.,6,72,252,309,387,576], whereas its facilitatory effect occurs earlier and undergoes potentiation[e.g.,6,72,252,309,387,576].

Only few of the studies dealing with the effects of morphine on self-stimulation attempted to reverse the behavioral effects with opiate antagonists. When an opiate antagonist such as naloxone or naltrexone was pre-administered to, or co-administered with, morphine, all behavioral effects of morphine were blocked[71,213,568,691]. However, the opiate antagonist naloxone did not *reverse* the rate-increasing effects of morphine when administered on the peak of this facilitatory effect[252]. Together, these data strongly suggest that the sensitization of ICSS is *triggered* by morphine, but sustained by a neural mechanism outlasting opiate receptor activation. This conclusion is supported by the observation that the peak effect of sensitization occurs about three hours after morphine administration[e.g.,6,72,112,252,387,388,462], when the drug has been cleared from the organism by as much as 75 percent[e.g.,33,52,307].

The effects of nicotine on self-stimulation are generally similar to those of morphine. Low doses of nicotine increase ICSS[151,572] or have no effect[101,464,678]. High doses generally cause an initial depressant effect, followed by increased lever pressing[464,37,58,59,100,101,272,465,572] but exceptions were observed[306,732]. Repeated injections of nicotine produce tolerance to its depressant effects[37,58,59,100,272,306]. In contrast to studies of morphine, most nicotine studies failed to find clear sensitization of its enhancing effect either on rate or on threshold[37,58,59,100,272].

3. THE INADEQUACY OF THE ICSS PARADIGM FOR ASSESSING DRUG PROPERTIES

The facilitatory effects of nicotine on ICSS have been generally interpreted as evidence for its reinforcing effects[e.g.,17,37,100,272,299,300,306,732]. As we aim to show in the rest of this chapter, however, studies of ICSS are irrelevant to the issue of nicotine addiction, for several reasons. First of all, in spite of extensive research (mainly performed during the 1960s), the exact nature of ICSS is not understood. Secondly, the effects of certain drugs on ICSS, most notably the opiates, contradict observations made with self-administration. Thirdly, it is difficult, if not impossible, to separate drug effects on locomotion from those that purportedly involve mechanisms of reward. Finally, even the assumption that drug reward and ICSS share the same mechanism is questionable. As a result, the effects of drugs on ICSS lend themselves to multiple interpretations and cannot be used to determine whether or not nicotine, or any other drug, is reinforcing.

3.1 Differences between Natural Rewards and ICSS

There are crucial differences between the behavioral effects of "natural" reinforcers, such as food and water, and those of ICSS. These differences have been discussed in detail elsewhere[198], so we shall mention them only briefly.

One difference between lever pressing for ICSS and for natural rewards concerns satiation. With food or drink reward, animals will work until they are satiated. In contrast, with the exception of specific electrode placements[459], they do not seem to reach satiation for ICSS. A second difference involves the speed of extinction. Consider a procedure where a thirsty animal is trained to press a lever for water and is working at a constant rate. If the experimenter switches off the mechanism that provides the water, the animal will continue to press the lever, initially at a high rate and later at increasingly lower rates. Finally, as it apparently learns that the lever no longer provides reward, it will stop pressing altogether[510]. In contrast, animals that have learned to press for electrical brain stimulation generally stop pressing much more rapidly. In this study[593], rats that had made as many as 10,000 responses per 15-minute session for 15 to 20 days stopped pressing abruptly when the electricity was disconnected, showing no extinction curve at all.

Furthermore, Olds and Milner[460] and others[163,666,702] observed that some rats did not resume pressing at the beginning of a new daily ICSS session and would initiate lever pressing only following "priming" – frequent stimulation administered by the experimenter. Such overnight decrements do not occur with food reinforcement[458,702]. Spontaneous recovery with ICSS was impaired even when inter-trial intervals were as short as ten seconds[197]. Consistent with this is the observation that self-stimulation is poor in partial reinforcement schedules, when time intervals are imposed between rewards[69].

Finally, in contrast with natural rewards, the motivation of animals to engage in ICSS is increased by the electrical stimulation itself. This is evident when "priming" induces or increases the rate of self-stimulation[e.g.,142,157,198,424,460,520]. This phenomenon is not found with other rewards. "Pre-feeding" hungry animals or "pre-watering" thirsty ones will not increase lever pressing for these rewards.

3.2   Limitations of the "Pure Incentive" Account of ICSS

The observations summarized above are inconsistent with the 'pure incentive' theory of self-stimulation. If ICSS is that rewarding, why is it so easily extinguished? Why is spontaneous recovery so poor? Why is there a need for "priming?"

The 'pure incentive' theory encounters other problems as well. As discussed earlier, this theory asserts that lever pressing for electrical brain stimulation should increase in the presence of other rewards. The implication of this prediction is that ICSS should decrease in the presence of aversive states. In numerous studies, however, anhedonic manipulations have had the opposite effect. Water and food deprivation increased ICSS[e.g.,24,74,193,226] and slowed extinction[140,206]. In the same vein, loud noise, tail pinch, restraint stress, and sometimes also inescapable foot-shock have been observed to increase ICSS[28,141,335,336,413,414], depending on the site of electrode implant.

ICSS was also reported to increase following deprivation of REM sleep[660] or oxygen[11].

Studies of shuttle-box self-stimulation have provided direct evidence that ICSS is not a "pure incentive." In these experiments animals can switch continuous electrical stimulation on and off to a "reward area" (in the sense that Olds used the term) of the brain, by moving from one area of the shuttle-box to the other. In these studies, without exception, the animals shuttled back and forth, alternately switching the current on and off[e.g.,22,23,24,29,137,320,589,669]. The fact that the animals switched the current off demonstrates that, at some point, electrical stimulation of the brain had become aversive.

3.3   The "Homeostatic" Account of Self-Stimulation

An alternative explanation of ICSS[142,198] is based on homeostatic theories that were postulated earlier by learning theorists. It proposes that brain stimulation in "reward" areas, rather than eliciting 'pure reward,' simultaneously produces an aversive 'drive' and a reinforcing effect which reduces this drive. Thus, depending on its placement, electrical brain stimulation can produce simultaneously both hunger and satiation. Following a lever press for electrical brain stimulation, the drive to eat outlasts the sensation of satiation and 'decays' only after some time. Hence, the animal will press the lever again to reduce its hunger, only to feel hungry again as soon as the rewarding effects of the electrical stimulation wear off.

The "homeostatic" hypothesis accounts for many of the enigmatic observations that characterize ICSS. It explains why animals show rapid extinction: as soon as stimulation stops, the animal has no drive for pressing the lever any further. The same reasoning explains the lack of spontaneous recovery following even short inter-trial intervals, and the need for 'priming' becomes obvious. In the same vein, food or water deprivation, or other anhedonic manipulations, increase ICSS by increasing drive. Finally, the theory explains the observation that animals in shuttle-box ICSS switch off electrical brain stimulation by postulating that electrical stimulation produces, over time, more drive than reward.

In addition, the homeostatic account is consistent with another well-established phenomenon. When the experimenter delivers electrical current to the same electrodes that sustain ICSS, animals often respond with feeding, drinking or sexual behaviors[e.g.,75,111,271,281,400,419,428]. These "stimulus-bound" responses are readily explained by the homeostatic hypothesis: As electrical stimulation induces drive as well as reward, the animal responds with drive-reducing behavior.

The theory of Deutsch and Gallistel has been criticized primarily on two counts. First of all, findings in the ICSS paradigm tend to vary. Drive decay is not apparent in all animals, spontaneous recovery is sometimes seen, and priming is not always necessary[e.g.,342,352,497,638]. Secondly, animals often display ICSS-directed behavior: as mentioned above, conditioned place preference for electrical stimulation prompted Olds and Milner[460] to attempt ICSS in the first place. Moreover, early researchers have demonstrated secondary conditioning of ICSS to previously neutral stimuli such as tones[346,628]. It is difficult to reconcile these observations with the thesis that the only reward involved in ICSS is drive reduction.

3.4   Summary: The Theoretical Status of Self-Stimulation

As stated before, it is not within the scope of this book to explicate the nature of ICSS. Our goal is only to portray the debate concerning the nature of self-stimulation and its implications for our (in)ability to interpret the effects of drugs in this paradigm. The need to underscore this debate stems from the fact that the literature concerning the effects of drugs on self-stimulation largely ignores it. This neglect is not surprising, as the rationale for testing the effects of drugs on ICSS rests on the validity of the 'pure incentive' account. Consequently, the results of most studies of drug effects on ICSS are explained according to the logic of 'pure incentive' theories, concisely stated by Wise[719]: "*...drugs of abuse generally increase responding for brain stimulation reward; they do so by increasing the rewarding potency of the stimulation* (p. 321)." Only few studies have recognized that psychoactive drugs can alter responding for brain stimulation reward in another way, specifically, "*by attenuating concurrent aversive properties of stimulation*[385] (p. 75)."

The statements cited above illustrate the essence of the unresolved debate between proponents of the 'pure incentive' account[461,629]and the 'homeostatic' account[142,198]. If self-stimulation has an aversive (or 'drive') component, then psychoactive drugs can increase self-stimulation in two ways: either by increasing the reward component, or by decreasing the aversive component. This, by itself, complicates the interpretation of results obtained with psychoactive drugs on ICSS. Furthermore, if the drive state postulated by the homeostatic theories causes the release of neurotransmitters, then agonists of these transmitters could be expected to increase ICSS *without being rewarding*. Similarly, any antagonist to these neurotransmitters could be expected to reduce ICSS, yet be rewarding.

In view of the unresolved debate between the 'pure incentive' and 'homeostatic' theories, it becomes impossible to interpret the ICSS results with any confidence. However, in addition to this thorny problem, there is another reason to doubt the validity of ICSS as a model for testing the reinforcing properties of drugs. Specifically, as we show below, the conclusions drawn from ICSS often contradict those obtained with the self-administration paradigm.

4. MORPHINE IN SELF-ADMINISTRATION VS. ICSS PROCEDURES

Both the self-administration and the self-stimulation paradigms are used to assess the reinforcing properties of drugs. These two models, however, yield results that contradict each other on both the behavioral and the pharmacological level. The effects of opiates on ICSS can be summarized as follows:

1. Morphine-like drugs first decrease, and subsequently increase the rate of self-stimulation[e.g., 6,72,112,252,387,388,462].

2. With repeated exposures to morphine, the depressant effect undergoes tolerance, whereas the facilitatory effect undergoes sensitization[e.g., 6,72,252,309,387,576].

3. The sensitization of the facilitatory effect is not reversible by opiate antagonists[252].

4. The peak effect of sensitization occurs about three hours following morphine administration[e.g., 6,72,112,252,387,388,462], when morphine has been cleared from the organism by as much as 75 percent[e.g., 33,52,307].

The effects of opiates in intravenous self-administration paradigms can be summarized as follows:

1. Rats self-administer opiates readily[60,129,203,391,409,451].

2. Over a period of about 2-3 weeks, rats increase their intake of morphine or heroin as much as five-fold[60,391,451]. This phenomenon is believed to reflect increased tolerance to the rewarding effects of the drug.

3. Opiate self-administration is fully reversible by opiate antagonists[e.g.,84,409,410].

4. The peak effect occurs within minutes after injection. Self-administration studies report rates of more than five injections per hour[60,129,203,391,409,451,692], indicating that the effect of each injection wears off within twelve minutes or less.

These brief summaries highlight the central contradictions between the two paradigms. Judging by the effects of morphine on ICSS, morphine's reinforcing (rewarding) effects peak an hour after morphine's half-life, undergo sensitization, and are difficult or impossible to reverse with opiate antagonists. In contrast, according to the self-administration model, the rewarding effects of morphine appear almost immediately, undergo tolerance, and are readily reversible by opiate antagonists. As these observations cannot be reconciled, one model must be wrong.

Of the two paradigms, the self-administration findings are more consistent with morphine- and heroin-induced euphoria in humans. The rewarding action of opiates is rapid, as noted by Jaffe[311]: "*At any point in the course of withdrawal, the administration of a suitable opioid will completely and dramatically suppress the symptoms of withdrawal (p. 534).*" The euphoric effects of these drugs undergo tolerance, which causes the gradual increase in doses administered by veteran users: "*... the addict who is primarily seeking to get a "rush" or to maintain a state of dreamy indifference (a "high") must constantly increase the dose. In this way, some addicts can build up to phenomenally large doses (e.g., 2 g of morphine intravenously over a period of 2.5 hours without significant change in blood pressure, pulse rate or respiration) (p. 533)[311].*" Finally, the rewarding effects of heroin are readily and completely reversed by opiate antagonists[311]. From this comparison, it appears unlikely that the effects of opiates on ICSS reflect their rewarding properties.

We have seen, then, that the effects of morphine on ICSS are different in critical respects from the results obtained from the self-administration paradigm. In contrast, the effects of morphine and other drugs, including nicotine, on ICSS are intriguingly similar to the effects of the same drugs on locomotion. This resemblance may provide a clue for another possible interpretation of the effects of drugs on ICSS.

5.   THE SIMILARITY BETWEEN THE EFFECTS OF DRUGS ON ICSS AND ON LOCOMOTION

The effects of morphine on locomotion, like the effects of other behavioral depressants, vary according to dose and over time. Low doses of morphine (up to about 5 mg/kg), administered acutely, have stimulant effects on locomotion in rats[e.g.,209,401,512]. Higher doses suppress locomotion in a dose-related fashion[e.g.,467,663], followed by increased locomotion[697]. With repeated injections, tolerance develops to the suppressant effects of morphine on locomotion[e.g.,672], whereas the stimulatory effects are potentiated or 'sensitized' following repeated injections[672,673]. In general, the effects of morphine on locomotion are very similar to its effects on ICSS.

The marked similarity between the effects of morphine on ICSS and on locomotion suggests that the two types of behavior may share similar mechanisms. Specifically, several observations suggest that the sensitization of locomotion is triggered by the activation of specific opiate receptors, but sustained by different mechanisms. First of all, it does not undergo tolerance. Secondly, increased locomotion was observed during spontaneous or precipitated withdrawal[38,39,476– but see 584]. Thirdly, sensitization does not disappear following a morphine challenge 92 hours[516], 7 days[4,697] or, with a selective delta-opioid agonist, even 2 months[418] after morphine withdrawal. Fourthly, with the exception of one study[673], there is no evidence that the sensitization of locomotion can be reversed by opiate antagonists. As the antagonist in this study was injected one hour before the peak of sensitization, its results are not conclusive[F].

[F] There exist two major differences between the effects of morphine on locomotion and ICSS. First of all, low doses (up to 5 mg/kg) of morphine consistently produce increases in locomotion, whereas the effects of such doses on self-stimulation are less consistent.

Researchers have tended to disregard the decreased ICSS rates following morphine as resulting from non-specific effects such as motor retardation[e.g.,167]; at the same time they attribute rate-increasing effects to a specific motivational aspect of behavior. In view of the similarity between the effects of morphine on locomotion and its effects on ICSS, this interpretation seems to reflect a theoretical bias rather than a balanced consideration of the evidence. Objectively, both the inhibitory and the facilitative effects of morphine on ICSS can be interpreted either as effects on performance or on motivation, or both.

Like the effects of morphine, the effects of other drugs on self-stimulation can be effectively predicted from their effect on locomotion. In a recent review[719] (p.328), stimulants which facilitate spontaneous behavior topped the list of drugs that increase self-stimulation. The same review also listed (without referring to the problematic issues discussed above) morphine and heroin, and some of the hallucinogens (psychedelics), such as cannabis and phencyclidine (albeit on the basis of only a few studies). In contrast, depressants such as alcohol, barbiturates and benzodiazepines reduce rather than facilitate self-stimulation[719], whereas apomorphine, which is not self-administered by humans, enhances self-stimulation [719].

Nicotine, at least at low doses, stimulates locomotion in rats (for locomotion references, see Chapter 5). At higher doses a biphasic depressant/activating effect becomes apparent, culminating in ataxia and catalepsy at very high doses and followed by increased locomotion. With repeated injections, tolerance to the depressant effects develops rapidly. On the basis of these observations alone, we can predict that the effects of low to moderate doses of nicotine will enhance self-stimulation rates, whereas

---

Secondly, spontaneous or precipitated withdrawal increases locomotion[38,39,476–but see584], but generally decreases ICSS[e.g.,569,571– but see330]. These differences seem to imply a dissociation between locomotion and self-stimulation, but they may simply reflect the fact that locomotion and lever pressing are incompatible, especially in the presence of escape behavior (jumping). In a so-called "rate-independent" measure of ICSS reward (the current threshold for self-stimulation[167]), locomotion is excluded. Hence, only drug activation of lever pressing is measured. In these studies, thresholds for lever pressing are perfectly correlated (across studies) with morphine dose-related shifts in locomotion where locomotion is the sole dependent variable. When doses of morphine lower than 5 mg/kg were used, threshold reductions were observed[e.g.,300,308,345,570,671]. Higher doses increase the current threshold[e.g.,166,168,213,289,353,576,671].

higher doses will lead to a reduction in responding – at least until the sedative effects wear off. Thus, following either a long latency between the injection and the stimulation session, or by inducing tolerance by repeated administration, nicotine can be expected to increase self-stimulation rates. This, with few exceptions, has indeed been observed.

As in the case of morphine, most authors discarded nicotine's depressant effects on ICSS as a performance deficit, while viewing its rate-enhancing effects as motivational. This bias was probably the reason that most researchers did not include appropriate experimental controls to determine which process was actually operating. A noteworthy exception is the study by Clarke and Kumar[101] who incorporated a simple control in their paradigm. Using shuttle-box self-stimulation, they simply shut off the current. They found that "... *responding was increased by nicotine even when brain stimulation was not available ('time-out')* (p. 271)," thus demonstrating that nicotine's effect in this paradigm can be attributed to its activating properties.

6.   SUMMING UP: SELF-STIMULATION AND NICOTINE REINFORCEMENT

The self-stimulation paradigm suffers from theoretical and empirical problems that, despite its extensive use, have never been satisfactorily resolved. As discussed above, the two dominant accounts of ICSS contradict each other, and neither is satisfactory. The ambiguity regarding the nature of ICSS is sufficient to invalidate its use for determining the reinforcing properties of drugs, including nicotine. In addition, this application of ICSS cannot be justified on empirical grounds. The central findings that contradict this use of ICSS are as follows:

1.   Animals behave differently in pressing a lever for ICSS compared to pressing for natural rewards.
2.   Results from ICSS drug studies contradict results from self-administration studies.
3.   The effects of drugs on ICSS are similar to, and confounded with, their effects on locomotion.
4.   Not only rewarding drugs but also aversive stimuli and states can increase self-stimulation.

5. Many drugs, notably depressants and alcohol, do not screen as rewarding drugs with the ICSS paradigm.

Taken together, both theoretical and empirical considerations indicate that the rewarding properties of psychoactive drugs, including nicotine, cannot be inferred from their effects on ICSS.

7.   A NOTE ON NICOTINE AND DOPAMINE

For nearly two decades, there was little doubt that mesolimbic and mesostriatal dopamine release was equivalent to reward. This dominant view was expressed in the 'anhedonia' hypothesis, formulated by Wise and his co-workers[186,187,718,722], which proposed that these dopamine systems mediated pleasure. When dopamine antagonists are administered to animals, according to this hypothesis, *"all of life's pleasures – the pleasures of primary reinforcement and the pleasures of their associated stimuli – lose their ability to arouse the animal*[718](p. 52)." Thus, dopamine was believed to mediate the pleasure of food, sex, and drugs of abuse.

As the 'anhedonia' hypothesis essentially equated dopamine release with reward, it lent itself to a simple and foolproof test of the rewarding properties of drugs: if a drug produces an increase in dopamine, it must be rewarding. According to this criterion, nicotine was clearly rewarding, as it was consistently reported to increase release of dopamine in the nucleus accumbens[e.g.,98,211,303,490,501,521,578], apparently by exciting ventral tegmental neurons[e.g.,77,177,389,494,578].

Evidence accumulated in recent years, however, has unequivocally refuted the assumption that dopamine release equals reward. As Gray and his colleagues [230] stated, *"This evidence shows that unpleasant events such as foot-shock increase extra-cellular levels of dopamine in the nucleus accumbens, as measured, for example, by in vivo intra-cerebral microdialysis. (...) We believe, in the light of findings such as these, that there is no special relationship between dopamine release in the nucleus accumbens and positive reinforcement* (pp. 1548-1549)." Or, in the words of Berridge and Robinson[50]: *"There can be no doubt that behavior needed to actively **avoid an unpleasant outcome** is impaired as strongly by dopamine suppression as behavior directed toward a positive reward* (p. 348, emphasis in original)." Aversive events such as foot-shock[620], forced exercise[128], tail pinch stress[127], restraint stress[302,304] and others [for review, see329,558] have all been shown to increase dopamine release in the nucleus accumbens.

There is little agreement amongst current researchers on the role of dopamine in reward. It has been argued that dopamine release in the nucleus accumbens is correlated with the novelty of the stimulus[e.g.,201,522], the relevance of the stimulus[329], reward learning[e.g.,12,13,41,105,143,430,585,586,707], and "wanting" (but not "liking") an event in the "incentive salience" theory[50].

Again, it is not within the scope of this book to evaluate these theories. Our goal in this brief summary is only to stress that the observation that nicotine causes the release of dopamine in mesolimbic and mesostriatal structures does not prove that it has reinforcing properties. Rather, depending on circumstances, it may indicate that nicotine is aversive, or novel, or somehow involved in learning processes. As we argued in regard to drug-facilitated ICSS, dopamine release cannot be taken as a reliable indication that nicotine, or any other psychoactive drug, is rewarding.

Chapter 8

REINFORCING PROPERTIES OF NICOTINE IN HUMANS

1.   NICOTINE AS A PRIMARY REINFORCER

There seems to be a consensus among researchers of tobacco smoking, with only few dissidents, that nicotine is reinforcing for humans.   The following statements illustrate this consensus: *"The ability of nicotine to regulate mood and improve cognitive functioning can act as a strong reinforcer of tobacco dependence* (p.96)[369];" *"Studies in both animal and human subjects have shown that nicotine can function as reinforcer, albeit under a more limited range of conditions than with some other drugs of abuse* (p.2)[635];" *"Thus the principal virtue of nicotine is its ability to make people feel good* (p.572)[316];" *"Subjective effects such as pleasure or "liking," which are assumed to be related to the reinforcing effects of nicotine, have also been studied in humans and appear to be directly related to the actions of nicotine in the brain. (...) In addition to the direct reinforcing effects obtained from nicotine use, its administration results in modulation of mood, appetite, and energy metabolism, and it may provide relief from boredom* (p.744)[265]."   Such statements, formulated with varying degrees of certainty and often without reference to experimental evidence, are abundant in the nicotine literature.   But in reality, only a few studies have tested whether nicotine is reinforcing for humans, and the results of most of them contradict these statements. Of the few studies that appear to support them, none has included appropriate controls to rule out alternative explanations.

1.1   Methodological Problems in Human Studies of the Reinforcing Properties of Nicotine

Hughes et al.[295] elegantly exposed two problems in studying the reinforcing properties of nicotine in humans. Participants were habitual smokers who declared that they wanted to quit smoking and agreed to abstain from smoking for the duration of the study. In the first of three studies, participants were told that they would receive either nicotine or placebo gum. With these instructions, participants consistently self-administered the nicotine gum significantly more than the placebo gum. However, these experienced smokers demonstrated an excellent ability to distinguish between the gums, apparently on the basis of the nicotine gum's side-effects. Therefore, they may have preferred nicotine gum not because they liked its psychoactive effects, but rather because they believed it would be more helpful for them in overcoming craving. Studies 2 and 3 provided compelling evidence in support of this hypothesis. In Study 2, participants were told they would receive either the marketed nicotine gum or a new nicotine gum (the same placebo) that was as effective as the marketed gum but had fewer side-effects. In Study 3, the experimenters told the participants to expect more side-effects from the placebo than from the nicotine gum. In both studies, participants self-administered equal amounts of placebo and nicotine gum. Thus, the instructions given to the participants controlled whether nicotine would serve as a reinforcer.

These experiments highlight two important observations, which are crucial to studies of nicotine in human participants and to the interpretation of an extensive area of nicotine research. The first is that human participants will respond according to their beliefs; the second, that smokers can identify nicotine by its physiological effects or taste. A conclusion from these two observations is that nicotine can be expected to have significant placebo effects. Therefore, nicotine-free gum, patch, nasal spray, or saline injection may not constitute appropriate controls for the effects of nicotine.

Unfortunately, this conclusion failed to have any impact on subsequent research.

Another concern in studies of nicotine in humans is the choice of participants. Clearly, everybody would be convinced that nicotine is reinforcing if people who never smoked liked the sensations that accompany nicotine administration. The consistent result of all studies, however, is that regardless of the mode of administration, people who never smoked dislike the effects of nicotine[e.g.,184,341,448,454,481,508,560,621,626,653]. Alternatively, if nicotine "replacement" devices would satisfy smokers as much as smoking does (or at least as much as methadone satisfies opiate users), this would also be a convincing demonstration that nicotine is reinforcing. This is also not the case (see Chapter 11). Instead, what is considered evidence for the reinforcing properties of nicotine in humans is the finding that deprived heavy smokers like nicotine as compared to placebo (see below). This type of evidence, however, is much less compelling and requires careful controls for alternative explanations. There are two parsimonious alternative explanations for the euphoriant effects of nicotine in deprived smokers. The first is that deprivation produces a negative mood, which is improved by the placebo effect of nicotine (resulting from smokers' beliefs and expectations regarding the effects of nicotine). The second is that nicotine, a salient cue, becomes a secondary reinforcer in smokers by consistent temporal association with other rewards. Regrettably, none of the experiments we reviewed employed controls for either of these alternative explanations.

2. EVIDENCE FOR THE REINFORCING EFFECTS OF NICOTINE IN HUMANS

To evaluate nicotine's role as a reinforcer in humans, it must be administered to, or be self-administered by, human beings in the absence of other factors that could be reinforcing. Pure nicotine has been administered to humans by injection or self-injection (intravenous or subcutaneous), by intranasal spray, via the transdermal nicotine patch, and by nicotine chewing gum.

2.1   Self-Administration of Intravenous Nicotine

Under the promising title of *"Human Studies of Nicotine as a Reinforcer,"* the Surgeon General's report[665] (p. 192) mentions no less than six studies where humans self-administered intravenous nicotine. Its summary of the subject is stated rather unequivocally: *"These studies of i.v. nicotine self-administration demonstrated conclusively that nicotine itself can serve as an effective reinforcer in humans."*

How conclusive is "conclusive?" The same strong and reassuring word, you may recall, was used in the Surgeon General's report to describe the extremely problematic study of four squirrel monkeys[220]. Hence, we may be justified for pausing to take a close look at the reports on which the present "conclusive" statement was based.

Out of the six references cited in this section of the Surgeon General's report, three[214,215,216] were made public only as abstracts or presentations, making methodological critique impossible. Another paper[646] is a non-refereed book chapter, leaving only two refereed studies of nicotine self-administration in humans[264,266]. These two studies were published in consecutive issues of the same volume of *Pharmacology, Biochemistry and Behavior*. Apparently, the second paper was reviewed before the first one was published, which may explain the peculiar fact that the two articles overlap in content. Each article reports results from six participants, but two of these participants (KU and KO) were included in both articles; the second article simply repeats the results of these two participants, figures and all.

Thus, the two articles that form the legitimate basis for the Surgeon General's "conclusive" statement regarding nicotine self-administration in humans include a grand total of ten participants. More importantly, the two studies share with the squirrel monkey study[220] the same research group, similar methodology and unfortunately, equally poor standards of design and presentation of results. As in the monkey study, partial figures and ambiguous text replace statistical analysis. The authors selectively report only the data that support their conclusions and hide problematic results behind suggestive wording. We shall endeavor to back this harsh criticism with prominent examples, but readers are encouraged to form their own impressions by reading the original reports[264,266].

The basic methodology of these studies was this: Male cigarette smokers sat in a reclining chair for a varying number of 3-hour sessions. They were prevented from smoking one hour prior to each session and during the session itself. An operant panel equipped with two levers was placed next to the chair. According to a preset schedule, pressing a number of times on one of the levers resulted in an intravenous injection of nicotine or saline; the other lever had no programmed consequences. Following each session, participants completed various questionnaires regarding their experience during the session.

The title of the first report[266] was *"Cigarette Smokers Self-Administer Intravenous Nicotine."* Its conclusion, as stated in the Abstract, was as follows: *"Nicotine injections were taken in orderly patterns that were related to unit dose, whereas patterns of saline injections varied widely. Furthermore, the volunteers reported that nicotine produced subjective effects similar to those produced by administration of abused drugs such as morphine or cocaine."* As we shall see, neither the title nor the conclusion is justified by the data.

To begin with, the six participants in this study self-administered both nicotine and saline. The authors failed to report the complete data on the number of nicotine and saline injections self-administered by their participants. The partial data they do report, however, reveal that some of the participants administered at least as much saline as they did nicotine. One subject for whom the number of injections is reported (SK), self-administered 22 saline injections, compared to only 8 injections of nicotine at the 1.5 mg dose, 5 at the 0.75 dose and 5 at the 3.0 dose. How can these data be interpreted as evidence for nicotine self-administration? If anything, they suggest a preference for saline over nicotine, hence a more fitting title for this article might be *"Cigarette Smokers Self-Administer Intravenous Saline."*

But this title would be just as misleading. The participants in this study were no ordinary "cigarette smokers." Four of the six participants *"had histories of abuse of a variety of drugs including opioids, stimulants and sedatives* (p. 887)[266]." Using ex-addicts as participants for a nicotine study is a remarkable methodological decision. As we have discussed earlier, there is considerable evidence that injection of saline, or even an injection ritual, may be reinforcing in such participants[503,696]. What can possibly be generalized from the behavior of participants with documented history of multiple drug abuse? Certainly not that *"Cigarette Smokers Self-Administer Intravenous Nicotine!"* As a matter of fact, in the two participants without a history of drug abuse, "*nicotine suppressed self-administration rates to levels well below those maintained by saline* (p. 1022)[264]."

The instructions given to the participants were ambiguous: "*Subjects were informed that participation in the study required only that they remain seated in the test room and not smoke cigarettes. They were told that pressing the levers might result in the injection of nicotine but they were neither required nor encouraged to press the levers* (pp. 888-889)[266]." What else were the participants, all deprived smokers and most with history of drug abuse and dependence, supposed to do for three hours per day, three sessions per week, for six to twelve weeks? Dream about good science?

Moreover, there is a striking contradiction in relation to these instructions, which apparently escaped the reviewers of this article. After each session, subjects were asked to identify the drugs they had self-administered. According to the authors, "*All four subjects with histories of drug dependence (including cocaine abuse) identified the nicotine injections as cocaine* (p. 889)." This is rather puzzling. How could participants who were expressly informed that pressing the lever might result in *nicotine* injections identify the drug as cocaine? Obviously, if the drug-experienced participants indeed identified nicotine as cocaine, then the findings concerning the pattern of nicotine administration by these participants are completely irrelevant for ordinary smokers!

In both studies, the authors justify their claim for nicotine self-administration by arguing that, even though participants administered both nicotine and saline, "*nicotine injections occurred in regular patterns whereas saline injections occurred with wide variability in pattern and frequency both within and across subjects* (p.1022)[264]." This claim is not backed by any evidence. The only information provided by the authors is a figure displaying the pattern of nicotine injections, and even this figure is incomplete: for three of the participants, it shows only a "*representative session*." The information on the pattern of saline injections, which is critical for comparison with the pattern of nicotine injections, is even more scant – it is provided in a schematic drawing for only one of the participants, who happens to be one of those with history of drug abuse. Furthermore, the authors claim that their figure "*shows that number of deliveries was inversely related to amount of drug per delivery. For subject PE, number of deliveries were 25 at saline, 49 at 0.75 mg, 20 at 1.5 mg, and 10 at 3.0 nicotine per injection. In the third subject tested under such a procedure (SK), number of deliveries were 22 at saline, 5 at 0.75 mg, 8 at 1.5 mg, and 5 at 3.0 nicotine per injection* (p. 888)[266]." It takes an extraordinary amount of good will to see an inverse relationship in these numbers, even if one ignores the fact that they represent only two participants.

In their second study[264] the researchers explored several variations of the previous procedure. Each variation, in the best tradition of the squirrel monkey study[220], was applied to only one or two participants. These variations tended to make the results even less compelling than those produced by the first study. In one variation, two participants were faced with a pair of levers. Pressing the right lever produced a nicotine injection, as in the original procedure, whereas pressing the left lever blocked the next scheduled injection (injections were scheduled at 30-minute intervals). Under these conditions of choice, *neither subject pressed the right lever*; in other words, both participants were entirely successful in avoiding all scheduled nicotine injections!

In summarizing the results of the second study, the authors seem to acknowledge the lack of any consistent pattern in their findings. *"In some of the subjects, nicotine maintained higher overall rates of lever-press responding than saline suggesting that nicotine was serving as a positive reinforcer. In other subjects overall rates of responding during sessions, when nicotine was available, were lower than those when saline was available, suggesting that nicotine was serving as a punishing stimulus relative to saline* (p. 1022)[264]." And later: *"Clearly, the data are not consistent with descriptions of nicotine as consistently serving as a positive reinforcer or an aversive stimulus, or simply as a toxin lacking behavioral effects* (p. 1025)." This summary is a much better reflection of their findings than their earlier one, which stated, unaccountably: *"Our findings are that tobacco deprived cigarette smokers self-administer nicotine, and that nicotine has euphoriant properties similar to morphine and cocaine* (pp. 889-890)[266]." But even this account is more prudent than the preposterous "summary" of these studies in the Surgeon General's report[665], which claimed that these studies *"demonstrated conclusively that nicotine itself can serve as an effective reinforcer in humans* (p. 192)."

2.2   Intravenous and Subcutaneous Administration Studies

Intravenous or subcutaneous nicotine administered to non-smokers has not been demonstrated to produce pleasant effects, improved mood, or any other positive subjective changes[183,184,204,360,370,448,545,621]. In fact, several recent studies demonstrated that nicotine via these routes is aversive to non-smokers[184,448,621]. The only exception[325] involved ex-smokers who *"had enough past experience with tobacco to understand the symptoms of nicotine toxicity* (p. 205)" and the effect was not significant.

Even in smokers, the effects of intravenous or subcutaneous nicotine were sometimes not positive[45,184,204,371] or even negative[184,371]. Yet, positive effects were reported in a few studies[267,325,545,621]. In all of these studies, however, participants knew they were receiving nicotine injections. Therefore, the results can be attributed, at least in part, to the placebo effects of nicotine in experienced smokers. Unfortunately, none of these studies included effective strategies to neutralize, or even assess, participants' expectations regarding the effects of nicotine. In addition, as noted above, any positive responses to nicotine in experienced smokers could reflect learning, that is, secondary reinforcing properties that nicotine may acquire by association with other reinforcers, including, as we discuss later in this chapter, the sensory rewards of smoking.

2.3   Nicotine Gum

Reports on mood changes or other affective changes with nicotine gum consumption are more consistent than with nicotine injections. Following the administration of nicotine gum to non-smokers, *"All subjects complained of nausea, dizziness or anxiety to varying degrees* (p. 297)[454]." According to Hughes et al.[296], *"Never-smokers reported the most dysphoria from nicotine, ex-smokers were intermediate, and current smokers reported the least dysphoria from nicotine* (p. 153)." Only one study[259] reported that nicotine gum increased ratings on the MGB (stimulant/euphoriant) scale[244], but as these non-smokers simultaneously reported a reduction in desire for another dose, it is unlikely that even in this study nicotine gum enhanced positive mood. The fact that nicotine gum is not self-administered by non-smokers[292] is a strong indication that it is not reinforcing for this population.

In smokers the results are not markedly different. In most studies smokers either did not derive any positive effect from nicotine gum or reported actual aversion[250,296,354,445,447,488,554]. We found only one study that claimed that smokers experienced pleasure from nicotine gum[475].

Despite the fact that nicotine gum is not associated with positive effects in smokers, many studies demonstrated that it causes a mild reduction in the severity of smoking withdrawal symptoms (see Chapter 11 for a full discussion). In view of the observation that smokers can discriminate between nicotine gum and placebo[e.g.,295], this finding indicates that nicotine gum may simply be a better placebo than the designated one.

2.4 Transdermal Nicotine

Two studies[659,685] reported that transdermal nicotine improves mood in abstaining smokers. Other studies[185,347,491,626] did not observe mood changes in smokers. These results are intriguing, as there is abundant evidence that transdermal patches in smokers cause adverse reactions such as sleep disturbances, nausea and vomiting, tiredness and dizziness[e.g.,79,232,327,617], which might be expected to dampen participants' mood. In non-smokers, these symptoms are a major reason for dropping out of clinical trials testing the effects of transdermal nicotine on ulcerative colitis[e.g.,508,560,653,670].

The mood of normal non-smokers was either unaltered by nicotine patches[208,559] or changed for the worse[341,508,560,626,653]. As was the case for injected nicotine and nicotine gum, we did not find a single report of transdermal nicotine patches inducing pleasure or improving mood in non-smokers (one study[379] reported increased vigor in non-smokers, with no additional mood changes).

3. NICOTINE DELIVERY KINETICS AND ABUSE LIABILITY

The following statements summarize the results of studies that examined the hedonic effects of nicotine, whether injected or administered by gum or transdermal patches. First of all, not a single study demonstrated that non-smokers enjoy nicotine. This finding may not have much significance, as most psychoactive drugs appear to be disliked by the novice. The next statement, however, is rather significant: In smokers, nicotine was found to be pleasurable in only four of eight injection studies, one of eight gum studies, and two of six patch studies – only 7 out of 22 studies altogether.

The extent to which the various modes of nicotine administration, including cigarettes, are pleasurable to smokers appears to correlate with the speed in which nicotine reaches the brain with these different devices. This hypothesis was formalized by Henningfield and Keenan[265] in a review titled *"Nicotine Delivery Kinetics and Abuse Liability."* The rationale for this hypothesis was based on evidence that rapid delivery of cocaine improves its subjective effects. This, apparently, is also true for heroin. Although many heroin addicts submit to methadone treatment, they prefer heroin and some continue to experiment with that drug during the initial months of methadone treatment[358]. Methadone is given orally, and its slow absorption does not provide the addict with the reportedly orgasm-like rush that accompanies heroin injection[311].

The generalization of findings from cocaine and heroin to nicotine, a distressingly common practice in nicotine research, is very problematic. It relies on the assumption that these drugs are similar in their mode of action and their role in maintaining the habits, which is exactly what must be established by research. Henningfield and Keenan[265] were aware of the paucity of empirical evidence for their hypothesis, noting that *"a single systematic study of nicotine delivery rate as a determinant of abuse liability has not been reported* (p. 743)[G]." Their own empirical contribution to the nicotine delivery hypothesis, however, is far from persuasive. It is confined to a series of studies from their group at the Addiction Research Center (ARC) of the National Institute on Drug Abuse, some of which were never published. As in other reports we reviewed by this group, sample sizes were very small (6–10), no statistical tests were conducted, and the authors did not

---

[G]This statement is still accurate today. We found one study in monkeys[679] claiming that nicotine's reinforcing effect is a function of infusion speed. However, infusion speed was shown in this study to be highly correlated with blood nicotine level. Therefore, any effects of infusion speed in this study (and in all likelihood, in similar studies as well) are attributable to the activating effects of nicotine.

even provide means and variances: the data are presented only in a summary figure[(Fig. 3)]. Even so, an objective examination of this figure finds no support for the authors' hypothesis. According to the figure, smokers dislike nicotine gum, are indifferent to patches, but like intravenous nicotine, inhaled nicotine, cigarettes and smokeless tobacco. The difference in response to cigarettes, on the one hand, and to gums and patches, on the other, is consistent with the idea that the speed of absorption may contribute to subjective liking: with smoking, nicotine enters the blood (and therefore the brain) faster than with gums and patches. However, the figure also shows that inhaled nicotine (from "smokeless cigarettes") is liked just as much as smoked nicotine, a fact that plainly contradicts the delivery kinetics hypothesis. As the authors themselves note, the smokeless inhalation method results in "negligible" nicotine absorption (p. 745). This crucial anomaly did not deter the authors from concluding that the data support their hypothesis. They handle the anomaly by claiming that their figure shows that *"even a vapor inhaler system with poor nicotine bioavailability may still produce effects characteristics of an abusable substance. Presumably, the inhalation route optimizes the reinforcing effects of the substance through sensory stimulation* (p. 747)." This statement demonstrates a disturbing lack of objectivity, which, again, is all too common in this area of research. Any impartial researcher would conclude that the observed pattern disconfirms the delivery kinetics hypothesis. If liking can be determined by sensory stimulation, then the nicotine delivery hypothesis has no explanatory power. In fact, if the inhaler delivers negligible quantities of nicotine and yet is liked just as much as smoking, the most obvious conclusion is that nicotine may have no role at all in determining liking.

There are other problems with the nicotine delivery kinetics hypothesis, which are not addressed by the authors. The hypothesis does not explain why nicotine gum was frankly aversive to Henningfield and Keenan's participants, or why the same participants were indifferent to transdermal patches. It does not explain the inconsistency of the findings obtained in all nicotine "liking" studies. It does not explain why a rapid delivery nicotine system such as Premier (heating tobacco rather than burning it) was a commercial flop[265]. It certainly does not explain why never-smokers do not like nicotine in any form.

In reading Henningfield and Keenan's review, it is evident that the authors were committed to the nicotine addiction hypothesis and were reluctant to be confused by inconvenient empirical findings, not even their own. This attitude is also reflected in an earlier discussion in the same article of a finding that is clearly problematic for Henningfield and his colleagues at the ARC. We quote: "... *Ernster et al. (1990) found that approximately 33% of baseball players who actively use smokeless tobacco during the approximately 8-month training and playing season abstained during the off-season. Nevertheless, smokeless tobacco is highly addictive (USDHHS, 1986), and the possibility that it is less addictive than cigarettes may be as clinically relevant as the difference between falling from a 20- and a 16-story building. Other characteristics of smokeless tobacco, including bioavailability profile and sensory characteristics, appear to maximize its addictive potential* (cf.[268], p. 747)." The rhetorical sequence here is illuminating: Henningfield and Keenan were confronted with a finding that clearly contradicts the presumed addictive nature of smokeless tobacco. They downplay the significance of this finding using a suggestive metaphor (after all, death is death, right?), reiterating their claim that smokeless tobacco "nevertheless" is "highly addictive." Finally, citing their own work and blatantly disregarding Ernster et al.'s[165] findings, they proceed to discuss variables that "maximize" chewing tobacco's "abusive potential." There is not even a pretence of scientific objectivity in this paragraph.

As is typical for this field, in which science, morals, and politics are hopelessly enmeshed (see Chapter 13), Henningfield and Keenan's hypothesis was uncritically accepted. It has become a popular truism in discussions of smoking, where cigarettes are described as an "*extremely effective nicotine delivery device*[e.g.,263]," "*providing nicotine 'hits' to the brain within seconds of smoke delivery to the lung*[657] (p. 93)." As we shall see later, delivery kinetics also became a popular fallback when researchers failed to find predicted patterns of nicotine self-administration or other indicators of addiction[e.g.,369,491]. This wide acceptance of the delivery kinetics hypothesis cannot be accounted for by its empirical basis. Moreover, the results of experiments with intranasal spray, a fast nicotine delivery system, are clearly inconsistent with the delivery kinetics hypothesis.

4.   STUDIES OF NICOTINE NASAL SPRAY

The observation that smokers are unenthusiastic about nicotine gum and patches can be explained in more than one way. The simplest explanation is that nicotine is not reinforcing for smokers and is far less important for maintaining the habit than is commonly believed. The explanation offered by the delivery kinetics hypothesis[265], however, was that the positive subjective effects of nicotine in smokers depend on rapid delivery of nicotine to the brain. It was therefore suggested that a nicotine nasal spray would be a more effective reinforcer than gums and patches, as nicotine absorption in the bloodstream following intranasal administration is nearly as fast as in smoking[for review, see581]. This hypothesis was not corroborated by research. Nicotine nasal spray was more effective than a placebo (a non-nicotine nasal spray) in three double-blind trials of smoking cessation[280,582,641], but none of these compared nasal spray to nicotine gum or transdermal patches. The only study known to us that compared nasal spray to nicotine gum and transdermal patches[246] concluded that "… *overall, there are no notable differences between the products in their effects on withdrawal discomfort, perceived helpfulness, or general efficacy* (p. 2033)."

The reinforcing effects of nicotine nasal spray have been remarkably well investigated by Perkins and his colleagues. Their studies found that, in smokers, nicotine-containing nasal spray either did not have significant positive effects on mood[479,480] or such mood changes were negative[481]. Consistent with all the nicotine administration literature, these authors also demonstrated that nicotine nasal spray has a more negative effect on mood[481] in never-smokers compared to non-smokers.

In two interesting studies, Perkins et al.[483,484] not only tested mood changes, but also let their participants self-administer nasal spray. In the first study[483], smokers were presented with two bottles of nasal spray. One colored bottle of nasal spray contained a nicotine solution, along with peppermint flavoring oil to disguise the nicotine taste and smell. The other bottle, in a different color, contained a placebo solution that, in addition to the peppermint oil, included pepper extract to control for the sensory effects of nicotine. Participants were asked to administer to themselves six sprays from each bottle, with a 15-minute rest between bottles. Subsequently, they were instructed to self-administer a total of six sprays from either or both bottles within a 3-minute period. This forced choice procedure was repeated every 15 minutes for 2 hours, for a total of eight trials. Participants participated in two afternoon sessions, one following overnight smoking abstinence and the other following no abstinence. Under the abstinence condition, participants self-administered equal amounts of the two sprays, thus demonstrating no preference for nicotine. Under the no abstinence condition, they self-administered *significantly less* nicotine nasal spray than non-nicotine spray. We interpret these results as showing that nicotine was neutral for deprived smokers and aversive for non-deprived smokers. The authors, however, interpreted these same data differently. They argued that the results support the role nicotine plays in smoking, as "*overnight tobacco abstinence was shown to significantly increase choice of nicotine...* (p. 262)." They address the lack of preference for nicotine over placebo, even in abstinent smokers, by arguing that this finding "*is perhaps consistent with other evidence that, in addition to nicotine's central effects, sensory effects from nicotine and non-nicotine constituents of smoking may contribute to smoking reinforcement*" (p. 261). In addition, they appeal to the delivery kinetics hypothesis[265] critiqued above, suggesting that "*reduced preference for nicotine spray vs. cigarettes may have been due to slower speed of nicotine delivery via spray* (p. 261)." Both of these explanations, however, are simply irrelevant to the finding that nicotine was never reinforcing in this paradigm and was unequivocally aversive to the non-deprived smokers. An obvious alternative explanation is that nicotine is simply not reinforcing for humans, a possibility that is well supported by evidence. But Perkins and colleagues, like most other researchers in this field, begin with the *premise* that nicotine is reinforcing for humans. Therefore, if findings appear to contradict this premise, these findings must be explained away. The belief that nicotine is reinforcing seems to be what Lakatos[363] called the "hard core" of this research program; it is simply not refutable by empirical evidence.

A later study by the same group, using a similar procedure[484] replicated the earlier study in that self-administration of nicotine nasal spray by smokers was not significantly different from chance (50%). In addition, self-administration of nicotine by never-smokers was *significantly lower* than chance, as it was for non-deprived smokers in the earlier study. Thus, the impartial conclusion from the two studies that examined self-administration of nicotine nasal spray can be summarized as follows: (1) Nicotine was aversive to never-smokers and to non-deprived smokers; (2) nicotine was not reinforcing to any participant group, including deprived smokers.

5.   SENSORY REWARDS IN SMOKING

The rewards of habits that involve drugs are not limited to the direct pharmacological effects of the drug on the brain. This is especially clear in the case of alcoholic beverages, as we discussed earlier. Humans spare no efforts in improving the taste of their wine, beer, and liquor. Aging of wines, blending of whiskeys, production of strengthened sweet wines like port and vermouth, adding sugar and herbs to liquor to create exotic liqueurs – all these practices have acquired the status of an art. There is no doubt that taste and smell contribute significantly to the pleasure of drinking, perhaps (especially in connoisseurs) even more than the reinforcing properties of the psychoactive agent, alcohol.

The consumption of tobacco is a behavior of an extraordinary complexity. Although some humans chew tobacco, particularly in the USA, most prefer to smoke it. Smoking often involves a preparation ritual (pipe cleaning, cigar moistening and cutting, the rolling of cigarettes), lighting, and ritualistic manipulation of the smoking material. As discussed earlier, rituals carry considerable weight in other habits involving drugs[189,503,696]. The contribution of such behaviors to the pleasure smokers derive from cigarettes and hence to the maintenance of the smoking habit was never systematically investigated.

Similarly, smoking produces extensive sensory stimulation. Oral stimulation, smell and taste, irritation of the mouth, upper airways and lungs may all contribute to the satisfaction humans derive from their habit. Experimental evidence shows that the relative contribution of sensory stimulation to smoking can hardly be overestimated.

5.1   Oral Stimulation

Perhaps due to the dominance of the nicotine addiction hypothesis, very little empirical work has been carried out to investigate the importance of oral stimulation for the satisfaction derived from smoking. It is well established that humans have a basic need for oral stimulation. Human fetuses have been reported to suck their thumb[270], demonstrating that this need is normal in early development. The soothing effect of oral stimulation in babies has also been extensively documented. Providing babies with a pacifier induces self-calming[188,525] and reduces crying, both in general[56,614] and in response to pain[80,81,240,323,422]. The use of the pacifier also has negative effects. It decreases social interaction and may lead to early termination of breast-feeding[188]. As the child grows up, the use of the pacifier becomes socially unacceptable, leading parents to embark on a struggle to wean their toddlers of this frowned-upon device. Removing the pacifier often causes irritability, crying and insomnia, symptoms that have motivated child psychologists to design effective methods of pacifier weaning[188]. Curiously, these "pacifier withdrawal symptoms" are similar to those observed following smoking cessation in adults[10].

The need for oral stimulation may persist through adulthood[87], but behaviors designed to satisfy this need are usually considered socially unacceptable. Society is not consistent in these matters: although it condemns thumb sucking and nail biting, it approves of other oral habits such as chewing gum. Thumb sucking and finger- or nail-biting, as unwanted habits, have been documented in hundreds of scientific publications[for review,see 485]. These behaviors may persist despite adverse consequences such as bleeding, deformed fingers and protruding teeth. Because of their obstinacy, these habits are often treated by professionals, often with similar behavioral techniques as are used for smoking cessation[e.g.,485,656,700,708]. In the same vein, commercially available 'plastic cigarettes' are often used as aids for smoking cessation. The relevance of oral stimulation to smoking was also demonstrated by a recent study[106], in which nicotine-free, normal chewing gum reduced craving for cigarettes in smokers.

Oral auto-stimulation, then, which starts at the pre-natal stage and is universal at infancy, may be habit-forming and persist into adulthood. Clinical psychologists and psychiatrists, notably Sigmund Freud, considered it a necessary phase in the development of human behavior. Whether one accepts this view or not, it is uncontested that oral habits, which do not involve self-administration of chemicals, can develop into compulsive behaviors that require professional help to terminate. The similarity between these observations and what is known about cigarette smoking suggests that oral auto-stimulation may significantly contribute to the prevalence and persistence of smoking.

5.2   Other Sensory Effects of Smoking

In 1977, Kumar et al.[359] demonstrated that when smokers inhaled tobacco smoke in the laboratory, subsequent *ad libitum* smoking was reduced in a dose-related way. In contrast, when comparable amounts of nicotine were administered intravenously, they failed to affect subsequent smoking. The authors concluded (p.528): *"Our negative findings, therefore, reopen the question whether physiologic dependence upon nicotine really is the basis for the tobacco-smoking habit. Is it possible that there is some other rewarding constituent of tobacco smoke?"* Subsequent experiments demonstrated that the answer to this question was affirmative.

Cigarette smokers often report enjoying the distinctive sensations in the respiratory tract that accompany each inhalation of smoke[19], sensations that are perceived primarily in the trachea[76]. This effect is caused principally by "tar" [541], but nicotine is also known to irritate oral and nasal mucosa [138,317] [233,297,314], an effect that can be blocked by the nicotine antagonist, mecamylamine[139,317].   The observation that nicotine has both central (psychoactive) and peripheral (sensory) effects, both of which are mediated by nicotinic receptors and can be blocked by mecamylamine, makes it difficult, if not impossible, to attribute observations to either way of action. For example, several studies that manipulated the nicotine yield of experimental cigarettes[48,152,170,221,242,249,590,723] found that nicotine yield determined subjective ratings or smoking patterns of these cigarettes (but see Grant et al.[229]).   However, the participants in these studies may well have reacted to the sensory effects of nicotine rather than to its central effects. Similarly, studies that used nicotine antagonists to manipulate the subjective effects of nicotine or smoking patterns[446,500,538,542,634] cannot rule out the possibility that their results reflect blockage of peripheral rather than central effects (see Scherer[577] for review and more detailed comments).

The importance of the sensory stimulation of "tar" for determining smoking patterns has been demonstrated in various ways. Sutton et al.[645] studied the relation of cigarette yield of nicotine, tar, and carbon monoxide to puffing patterns and blood concentrations of nicotine, using a sample of smokers who smoked their usual brand of cigarettes. They found that the tar yield of the cigarettes determined puffing patterns (and hence blood levels of nicotine) to a much higher degree than nicotine. *"When nicotine yield was controlled for, smokers of low-tar cigarettes not only puffed more smoke*

from their cigarettes than smokers of higher-tar cigarettes but they also had
higher plasma nicotine concentrations, suggesting that they were
compensating for the reduced delivery of tar by puffing and inhaling a
*greater volume of smo*ke (p. 600)." Stepney[630] had smokers of medium
nicotine/medium tar cigarettes switch to either low tar/medium nicotine or
low tar/low nicotine cigarettes. He found that both low tar cigarettes were
"oversmoked," resulting in significantly higher nicotine blood levels in
smokers of low tar/medium nicotine cigarettes compared to their regular
brand. In several subsequent experiments using experimental cigarettes of
varying tar and nicotine yield, smoking patterns did not depend on the
nicotine yield of the cigarettes[57,533,680] or depended on tar rather than nicotine
yield[26,255,411,529].

Just like smoking patterns, subjective ratings of satisfaction, pleasantness,
harshness and desirability were unrelated to nicotine content of cigarette
smoke[57,533] or depended on "taste" rather than on nicotine[310,450]. Cigarettes
equal in tar but higher in nicotine yield were rated as more satisfying, more
enjoyable and stronger in various experiments[25,26,255], but these experiments
did not control for nicotine's peripheral sensory action.

Several of the studies cited above showed that cigarettes that were low in
or devoid of nicotine suppressed withdrawal symptoms in nicotine-deprived
smokers[25,26,255,699]. In one study of particular interest[73], the investigators
provided smokers with denicotinized ("de-nic") cigarettes (.09 mg nicotine
and 10.8 mg tar) and compared their effects with those of regular cigarettes
(containing 1.1 mg nicotine and 15.9 mg tar). Denicotinized cigarettes
suppressed withdrawal symptoms just as well as regular cigarettes, despite
the fact that they did not increase plasma nicotine levels. As the authors
acknowledged, these findings *"support the importance of sensory factors in
the maintaining of smoking behavior and tobacco withdrawal* (p. 96)."

Other lines of evidence also support the contribution of sensory
stimulation of the airways to smoking satisfaction. Withholding sensory
stimulation by partial anesthetization of upper and lower airways in heavy
smokers resulted in significantly decreased craving for cigarettes[543]. This
decrease was correlated with the extent of the anesthesia, and reduced
craving by over 40 percent. Conversely, supplying smokers with sensory
stimulation, similar to that produced by cigarette smoke, is sufficiently
rewarding to reduce smoking and craving for cigarettes[381,535,540]. In these
experiments, the investigators had smokers self-administer puffs of citric acid

aerosol that irritates the respiratory system. Participants were asked to compare the subjective pleasure and satisfaction they derived from this aerosol to puffs of air, low tar and nicotine cigarettes, or the smoker's own brand. In these studies, citric acid aerosol reproduced some of the subjective pleasure and satisfaction associated with smoking. Participants liked the puffs of citric acid better than the control puffs of air and better than the low tar and nicotine cigarette. Moreover, after receiving several puffs of citric acid, reported satisfaction was higher and residual desire for a cigarette was lower than after control presentation of air. This effect equalled or surpassed that of the low tar and nicotine cigarette[540]. Rose et al.[535] concluded that *"subjects regulated their smoking behavior to equate sensory intensity rather than nicotine intake* (p. 891)." Along the same lines, Westman et al.[701] found that citric aerosol increased success rate in a smoking cessation trial.

5.3 Nicotine Nasal Spray Revisited: Effect of Nicotine on the Brain or Sensory Stimulation?

Nicotine nasal spray was found to be more effective than a placebo in three placebo-controlled, double-blind trials of smoking cessation[280,582,641]. Although this effect could be attributed to the action of nicotine on the brain, these studies did not test the extent to which sensory stimulation of the throat (which were reported by 73–100 percent of the participants) was responsible for this effect. In fact, there is good reason to suspect that sensory stimulation is a major factor in the effectiveness of nicotine-containing nasal spray on smoking reduction. We have shown above that specific sensory stimulation, which imitates the sensations produced by cigarette smoking, can significantly reduce craving in smokers. More specifically with regard to nasal spray, we discussed two studies by Perkins et al.[483,484] in which several groups of participants, both smokers and non-smokers, significantly preferred non-nicotine pungent spray to nicotine spray and no group, including abstinent smokers, showed preference for nicotine.

A comparison[506] of two studies that examined blood levels of nicotine following its administration further corroborates the contribution of sensory stimulation to the effects of nicotine nasal spray. Conze et al.[109] reported that a buccally administered nicotine solution, producing an increase in blood nicotine of approximately 10 ng/ml, had no effect on short-term, *ad libitum* smoking behavior. Perkins et al.[482], in contrast, reported that nicotine nasal spray, which produced the same increase in blood nicotine of roughly 10 ng/ml, did suppress *ad libitum* smoking behavior. These findings led the authors to conclude that "*smoking behavior is partly influenced by factors other than nicotine regulation* (p. 627)." These other factors, according to the converging evidence we have reviewed, consist in large part of sensory stimulation of the mouth, upper airways and lungs.

6.   CONCLUSION

At the beginning of this chapter we cited several researchers who stated, with various degrees of certainty, that nicotine is reinforcing in humans. We found almost no empirical support for this statement. On the contrary, research shows that people do not enjoy nicotine injections, gums, patches, or intranasal spray and many suffer from symptoms such as nausea and vomiting, headaches and sleep disturbances. Nearly all nicotine administration studies, regardless of the route or speed of delivery, indicate that nicotine is aversive to naive participants. In smokers or ex-smokers, nicotine is generally less aversive. This difference may be attributable to an acquired tolerance in smokers to the aversive effects of the drug, an issue we shall re-address in discussing the "compensation" hypothesis (see Chapter 12).

Our review of the evidence provides a solid basis for concluding that the sensory stimulation produced by cigarette smoking is reinforcing to smokers. In contrast, the evidence for nicotine having similar reinforcing properties is very weak. A minority of studies found that nicotine can be reinforcing for abstaining smokers. The most parsimonious explanation for this observation relies on the fact that in these studies, nicotine was discriminated from the intended placebo by its physiological effects[295,479,480,484]. Once recognized, nicotine can be experienced as pleasurable and relieve craving for smoking by two related mechanisms (a third possible mechanism, namely that nicotine is a negative reinforcer for humans, is ruled out by experimental evidence, as we shall show in the next chapter). First, smokers expect nicotine to relieve craving, an expectation that may give rise to a placebo effect, as discussed earlier. Second, nicotine can become a secondary reinforcer through repeated paring with other rewards. These include not only the pleasurable taste, smell, sensory and oral stimulation that smoking provides directly, but also rewards that are associated with smoking. One such reward is social reinforcement, which has been shown in several publications to be an important determinant of smoking[332,404,417]. Other rewards are the pleasurable states that can become associated with smoking, such as having coffee or alcoholic drinks, relaxing after a meal or sexual activity.

We want to remind the reader of the three primary criteria of drug addiction the Surgeon General deemed sufficient to define drug dependence. These criteria were "highly controlled or compulsive use," "psychoactive effects," and "drug-reinforced behavior." According to all available evidence, the self-administration of pure nicotine, in whatever mode of delivery, does not meet these primary criteria for drug addiction. Even deprived heavy smokers hardly self-administer pure nicotine; they certainly do not do it in a "highly controlled or compulsive" way. The psychoactive effects of nicotine are mostly adverse, and clearly do not constitute a motivation for further self-administration. In fact, we found no credible evidence that nicotine is more desirable to humans than saline. In summary, the research we have reviewed in this chapter provides no empirical basis for the universally accepted claim that smoking is maintained by the positive reinforcing psychoactive effects of nicotine.

Chapter 9

TOLERANCE TO AND PHYSICAL DEPENDENCE ON NICOTINE

Tolerance to a drug is defined as the need for an increased dose following long-term consumption in order to obtain the same effect or diminished effect with continued use of the same amount. Physical dependence on a drug is defined as the appearance of a characteristic withdrawal syndrome following drug cessation. Tolerance and physical dependence were the hallmarks of addictive drugs according to the classic definition discussed in Chapter 2. With the historical changes in the definition of addiction, these criteria are no longer required, and appear only as "tertiary criteria" in the Surgeon General's[665] definition. Despite this change in status, these phenomena merit detailed discussion. If tolerance to the reinforcing effects of nicotine (if these exist) could be demonstrated, and nicotine abstinence following long-term use could be shown to effect a nicotine-specific withdrawal syndrome, nicotine would be considered addictive even according to the most conservative definition of the term.

1. DEMONSTRATING TOLERANCE TO THE REINFORCING EFFECTS OF DRUGS

As mentioned before, psychoactive drugs produce many effects, only a few of which constitute reasons for which these drugs are self-administered by humans and animals. It is widely assumed that psychoactive drugs are self-administered because of their ability to produce euphoria, operationally defined as reinforcing effects. This is what the DSM refers to as the "*desired effect* (p. 176)[10]" of drugs. Most drugs also produce physiological effects that are neutral in terms of their reinforcing value. Nicotine, for example, elevates heartbeat and blood pressure and reduces appetite. Some effects of psychoactive drugs are frankly aversive, as was demonstrated in animals using conditioned taste aversion paradigms. Nicotine, for example, can produce nausea and vomiting even in regular smokers[e.g.,131,327]. As only the reinforcing (rewarding, euphoric) effects motivate self-administration of psychoactive drugs, it is irrelevant to demonstrate that the neutral effects of a given drug undergo tolerance. While such tolerance may well develop, it has no bearing on self-administration. The crucial question is whether the *reinforcing* effects of the drug undergo tolerance.

There are two ways of answering this question affirmatively. The first is to demonstrate that humans and animals will self-administer increasingly higher doses of the drug over time. This is well established for the opiates, for example, where animals were shown to self-administer increasingly higher doses over time[e.g.,60,391,451]. Although the development of opiate tolerance was partially confounded by the simultaneous acquisition of operant behavior in these studies, tolerance is evidenced by the fact that opiate-dependent and post-dependent animals self-administer higher doses of heroin than non-dependent animals[129]. In humans this question is more difficult to address, as addicted individuals are only rarely given the opportunity to self-administer unlimited quantities of opiates. Under normal circumstances, the amounts of heroin or morphine that opioid-dependent individuals self-administer are restricted by the prohibitive prices of the black market. Nevertheless, "… *if the drug is used frequently, the addict who is primarily seeking to get a "rush" or to maintain a state of dreamy indifference (a "high") must constantly increase the dose. In this way, some addicts can build up to phenomenally large doses (e.g., 2 g of morphine intravenously over a period of 2.5 hours without significant change in blood pressure, pulse rate, or respiration) (p.533)[311].*" Note that tolerance, in this description, pertains specifically to the euphoric effects (the "rush" or the "state of dreamy indifference") of heroin.

Yet, increased self-administration is not sufficient to demonstrate tolerance to the reinforcing effects of most drugs. There is an alternative explanation for the findings that drug-dependent humans and animals increase drug intake over time. Most, if not all, psychoactive drugs have aversive as well as euphoric effects and these aversive effects may limit the dose animals or humans are willing to self-administer. If the aversive effects of the drug undergo tolerance, the addicted animal or person can gradually increase drug intake. The most persuasive evidence for the proposition that the euphoric, rather than the aversive, effects of the drug undergo tolerance is to demonstrate that the increase in drug self-administration over time continues after tolerance to the aversive properties has already been established.

2. TOLERANCE TO THE EUPHORIC EFFECTS OF NICOTINE

There is little doubt that some effects of nicotine undergo both acute and chronic tolerance[for review, see 665, pp. 47-52]. In humans, acute tolerance (minor increment with successive injections of nicotine) has been demonstrated to arousal level, heart rate, and blood pressure[46,545]. Acute tolerance has been demonstrated to the lethal dose of nicotine in mice[34], to the dose that depresses locomotion in rats[632] and to a variety of other behavioral and physiological effects[for review, see 631]. Chronic tolerance in animals has been demonstrated to nicotine effects on locomotion[e.g.,633], operant responding[e.g.,262], EEG[288], and a variety of endocrine responses[for review, see 665].

Thus, both acute and chronic tolerance develops to a wide variety of the behavioral and physiological effects of nicotine. This is not surprising, as many drugs share this feature, including some that are not voluntarily self-administered by either animals or humans[311]. In contrast, not a single instance of tolerance to the euphoric effects of smoking, as evident from increased self-administration over time, is provided in the Surgeon General's[665] report, either in humans or in animals. This, too, is not surprising, as evidence for such increased intake of nicotine over time is simply not to be found in the literature even 12 years following this report. On the contrary, it is well-established that humans actually reduce nicotine-intake over time (see Chapters 10 and 12).

We could not find any animal studies that systematically investigated whether or not tolerance to the reinforcing effects of nicotine occurs. Whenever increases in lever pressing rate over time were reported, they were attributable to the activating effects of nicotine (see Chapters 5 and 6).

2.1   Do Humans Develop Tolerance to the Euphoric Effects of Nicotine?

When people start smoking, they reach the level of their preferred number of cigarettes quite rapidly, and this number tends to remain stable over the years[665, Table 9, p. 579]. The rapid initial increase of smoking could constitute evidence for tolerance to the euphoric effects of nicotine, but several lines of evidence contradict this interpretation.

First and foremost, there is strong evidence that the increase in cigarette consumption is caused by increased tolerance to the aversive, rather than to the reinforcing, effects of nicotine. Chronic tolerance to the aversive effects of nicotine in humans was demonstrated in experiments showing that nicotine produces more nausea in non-smokers than in smokers[e.g.,184] and less in ex-smokers compared to never-smokers[508]. This tolerance is not complete: nausea reappears when smokers increase their normal tobacco consumption by 50 percent[131]. Secondly, as we showed in Chapter 8, nicotine is not reinforcing in non-smokers, so its weak reinforcing properties in smokers must be learned. This learning process coincides with the initial period of smoking and produces the same outcome as tolerance to reinforcing effects would produce, namely an increase in the consumption of cigarettes. Thirdly, the hypothesis that the initial increase in cigarette consumption reflects tolerance to the reinforcing properties of nicotine cannot account for the observation that this trend does not continue over the lifetime of smokers. In fact, after the age of 55, cigarette consumption tends to decrease over time[665 Table 9 and 10, p. 579].

It could be argued that further increases in smoking are impossible because of incomplete tolerance to the toxic effects of nicotine. In other words, smoking of a certain number of cigarettes elevates blood levels of nicotine to an absolute ceiling beyond which nicotine-induced nausea prevents further increase. There is some evidence for this proposition (see Chapter 11 for a detailed analysis), but nicotine satiation does not seem to be the only factor that restrains increased smoking. The average nicotine yield of commercial cigarettes has decreased three-fold since 1954, from 2.7 mg/cigarette to 0.9 mg/cigarette in 1992[283,665]. If nicotine toxicity were the only factor that restrained smokers, the average number of cigarettes smoked should have increased threefold since 1954. As far as can be gleaned from available epidemiological evidence from the USA, this has not been the case[449].

In addition, surveys commonly find that 10–18 percent of smokers smoke five or fewer cigarettes per day and do so for many years without increasing their intake[247]. These smokers have been labeled "chippers[598]." Studies comparing chippers to heavy smokers found that chippers' intake of cigarettes over the years, while smaller, is just as stable as that of heavy smokers. At the same time, chippers were reported to have the same sensitivity to the physiological effects of nicotine as heavy smokers[599]. As the smoking pattern of chippers cannot be explained by an absolute ceiling imposed by nicotine's toxic effect, non-pharmacological factors must be involved in the regulation of smoking. We shall speculate on these factors in Chapter 12.

In conclusion, there is simply no evidence of tolerance to the reinforcing effects of nicotine in humans or animals. The initial increase in cigarette consumption when smoking begins is most likely related to increased tolerance to the aversive properties of nicotine, perhaps conjoined with the process by which smoking, and possibly also nicotine, acquires secondary reinforcing properties. The subsequent stability in cigarette consumption, together with the reduction in smoking that occurs in older smokers, indicates that smokers do not develop tolerance to the euphoric effects of nicotine.

3. PHYSICAL DEPENDENCE ON HEROIN

In opiates, precipitated withdrawal (by administering an opiate antagonist such as naloxone or naltrexone) or discontinuation of administration is followed by a highly dysphoric abstinence syndrome, with characteristic time course and symptoms. This syndrome is a powerful negative reinforcer: The opiate dependent individual is highly motivated to avoid this syndrome or reduce its severity. In the words of Kreek (p. 557)[358]: *"What we learned was that the addict self-administers heroin three to six times each day, first to simply achieve a "high" or euphoric effect: in time, with the development of increasing tolerance, the addict needs to continually escalate doses of heroin self-administered simply to prevent the appearance of opiate withdrawal symptoms."*

Depending on interpersonal differences, similar dysphoric withdrawal symptoms may motivate the continued self-administration of other drugs[311]. The dysphoric nature of alcohol and opiate abstinence syndromes has been confirmed by numerous reports on human users[311]. At the same time, the opiate and alcohol withdrawal syndromes are clearly distinct from each other[311]; in other words, they are *drug-specific*. This distinction is corroborated by examining the "cross-dependence" between these drugs, namely, the ability of one drug to suppress the manifestations of physical dependence produced by the other without canceling the dependent state. Thus, partial cross-dependence exists between ethanol and other sedative-hypnotics, while heroin has cross-dependence only with other opiates that act on the same type of opiate receptor (e.g., methadone and morphine[311]). In addition, there are some overlapping symptoms (e.g., restlessness, irritability, insomnia, and craving) that are not specific to a particular drug. These common symptoms are attributable to the fact that the interruption of a chemical addiction is also the interruption of a compulsive habit (see Chapters 2 and 10).

Two lines of evidence demonstrate that the opiate withdrawal syndrome is also dysphoric in animals. Direct evidence for this assertion is provided by the observation that the opiate withdrawal syndrome can produce both conditioned taste aversion and conditioned place aversion[e.g.,442,443]. Indirect evidence for the dysphoric nature of opiate withdrawal in animals is elicited in the following experimental procedure. In the first phase, animals are trained to self-administer heroin intravenously by pressing a lever. When stable pressing rates are reached, the effective dose of heroin following each lever press is reduced – either by reducing the amount of heroin, or by injecting, simultaneously with the heroin, a low dose of a competitive antagonist. According to learning theory, if the amount of the positive reinforcer is reduced, animals should be less willing to work and should reduce the number of times the bar is pressed. However, the opposite actually happens: the animals now press the bar *more* frequently, thereby increasing the amount of heroin they self-administer[e.g.,169,276,343,350,444]. If the dose of heroin is now increased, the frequency of lever pressing will decrease, again contrary to the prediction of learning theory[549]. The probable explanation for these observations is that as a result of a reduction in the dose of heroin, the animals experience dysphoric withdrawal symptoms; in response, the animals work harder to maintain their heroin intake and avoid the withdrawal syndrome. In conclusion, the evidence reviewed above establishes that the opiate withdrawal syndrome is dysphoric for both animals and humans.

4.   THE "NICOTINE ABSTINENCE SYNDROME" IN RATS

Whereas withdrawal from nicotine in humans is typically tested with individuals who have self-administered nicotine for long periods, generally by smoking, this paradigm is not routinely employed with animals. Instead, two other paradigms have been used in animal research on nicotine dependence.

In the first paradigm, rats self-administer nicotine, following the operant conditioning procedures described earlier (Chapters 5 and 6). When stable levels of lever-pressing are reached, the experimenter injects the animals with the nicotine antagonist mecamylamine, after which subsequent lever pressing is recorded. In similar experimental conditions with heroin, the antagonist facilitates lever pressing at low doses and suppresses lever pressing at high doses (see previous section). In nicotine studies, in contrast, mecamylamine only suppressed intravenous self-administration in a dose-related fashion[220,406,527,601,623]. When an increase was reported in one study, it was not statistically significant[115]. Increasing the dose of nicotine after injecting mecamylamine did not restore self-administration in the only study where this was tested[623]. This is also in contrast to findings with heroin in a similar experimental design[549]. The lack of facilitative action of mecamylamine strongly suggests that blocking nicotinic receptors does not produce a dysphoric abstinence syndrome. Hence, animal studies indicate that precipitated withdrawal, a hallmark of physical dependence, cannot be produced in the case of nicotine.

In the second paradigm, nicotine is administered by the researcher, rather than by the animal. This is usually done by implanting an osmotic minipump in the animal that delivers nicotine at predetermined doses for a period of days or weeks. As in humans, nicotine administration can be terminated by either removing the pump (spontaneous withdrawal) or by injecting the nicotine antagonist, mecamylamine (precipitated withdrawal).

A "nicotine abstinence syndrome" in rats, reproducible in both spontaneous and precipitated behavioral procedures, was first reported by Malin and colleagues[394]. This syndrome resembles the behavioral signs of opiate withdrawal, including teeth-chattering, chews, abdominal writhes, gasps, ptosis, wet shakes, and tremors. Malin and his group replicated and extended this finding in subsequent studies[e.g.,392,395,396,397,398] as did other groups[5,277].

The nicotine abstinence syndrome is problematic in several respects. Firstly, the behaviors that are scored as components of the syndrome are also found in animals that are nicotine free[e.g.,5,277,394], sometimes in up to 70 percent of the frequency scored in animals with precipitated withdrawal[5,277]. Secondly, the behavioral observations are strongly influenced by experimenter expectations: the number of withdrawal signs scored in nicotine-free animals when they served as double-blind controls for withdrawal was more than double the number scored at baseline[394]. Thirdly, the nicotine antagonist mecamylamine, at a dose of 5 mg/kg, produced as many withdrawal signs in *nicotine naive* rats as a lower dose of this compound (1 mg/kg) produced in rats that were infused with nicotine continuously for seven days[392]. Sensitization of opiate receptors to opiate antagonists following long-term pretreatment with opiate agonists is a well-known phenomenon[e.g.,344]. If a similar phenomenon occurs in nicotine receptors, the nicotine abstinence syndrome could well turn out to reflect the direct effects of mecamylamine, rather than of nicotine withdrawal. Fourthly, the peripherally acting nicotine antagonist chlorisondamine[277] also precipitated the same syndrome, indicating that the withdrawal reaction may involve peripheral, rather than central nicotinic receptors. Finally, even if the behavior described by Malin and coworkers does constitute a genuine nicotine abstinence syndrome, there is no evidence that this syndrome is, in any way, dysphoric (see section 4.3 below). This is a crucial point, as without such evidence there is no reason to believe that this syndrome can act as a negative reinforcer to facilitate further drug consumption.

4.1 Is the Nicotine Abstinence Syndrome in Rats Relevant to Smoking?

The problems summarized above discredit the validity of the nicotine abstinence syndrome in rats. Even more importantly, this model is inconsistent with observations in humans.

First and foremost, while the nicotine abstinence syndrome in rats can be produced by administration of the nicotine antagonist mecamylamine, no study has successfully replicated this basic procedure in human smokers[e.g.,162,493].

Secondly, the nicotine abstinence syndrome in rats has been reported to resemble a weak opiate withdrawal syndrome. Moreover, the opiate antagonist naloxone precipitates nicotine abstinence symptoms in chronically nicotine-treated animals[5,393]. These findings indicate that the nicotine abstinence syndrome in animals may involve opiate receptors. In humans, the smoking abstinence syndrome does not resemble opiate withdrawal[10,311], and the effects of opiate antagonists on smoking are contradictory. Some investigators found that opiate antagonists decreased smoking[227,333,703], whereas others found no effect[446,472,640]. If endogenous opioids are implicated in smoking, however, opiate antagonists should produce an initial compensatory *increase* in smoking, as was reported for the nicotine antagonist mecamylamine[446,500,536]. Opiate antagonists produced negative mood changes in smokers in some studies[61,472,703] but had no effects on mood in others[227,333,446]. In one study, opiate antagonists reduced the perceived difficulty of abstaining from smoking[640]. However, whereas plasma nicotine levels were correlated with mood states during periods of chronic smoking, abstinence and treatment with "nicotine replacements" devices, changes in plasma beta-endorphin levels were not related to changes in mood. Thus, if nicotine withdrawal in humans involves endogenous opiate systems, the nature of this involvement remains unclear and the relevance of nicotine withdrawal in rats to human smoking withdrawal symptoms seems marginal at best.

The differences between nicotine abstinence in rats and humans are not unexpected. Whereas the abstinence syndrome in animals follows discontinuation of long-term administration of nicotine, the withdrawal syndrome in humans follows the discontinuation of *smoking*. Thus in humans, in contrast to rats, the syndrome follows the interruption of a habitual behavioral pattern. Moreover, the central features of nicotine withdrawal in humans, unlike those of opiate withdrawal, are subjective and can only be assessed with self-report measures. In animals, only observable measurements can be used, which makes it impossible to compare the two syndromes in a meaningful way. Taken together, these differences between the rat "nicotine abstinence syndrome" and human smoking cessation invalidate this syndrome as an animal model for nicotine withdrawal in humans.

4.2   Other Effects of Nicotine Withdrawal in Animals

In addition to the nicotine abstinence syndrome discussed above, other behavioral consequences of nicotine withdrawal in the rat have been reported. Chronic nicotine administration in animals, as in humans, reduces food intake and weight gain, and its discontinuation produces the opposite effect[e.g.,103,380,717]. Although these effects were not always found[e.g.,260,730], this discrepancy can partially be explained by dose differences[260].

Interestingly, whereas chronic nicotine exposure has a stimulant effect on operant responding[e.g.,121], withdrawal from chronic nicotine has been shown to disrupt complex operant behaviors[e.g.,27,85,121,182] but not simple ones[e.g.,260]. A related finding is that withdrawal following chronic nicotine administration enhances the response of rats to auditory startle[e.g.,260,261,514]. Together, these results suggest that nicotine withdrawal in animals is associated with increased arousal.

In addition to operant responding, there are other behaviors that are affected by acute nicotine administration but are not symmetrically altered by nicotine withdrawal. For example, low doses of nicotine in acute administration, as well as chronic administration of high doses of this drug, have stimulant effects on locomotion[e.g.,99,322,433,574]. However, the rate of locomotion following cessation of nicotine administration in rats is not reduced beyond control or baseline values[99,260,633].

4.3 Are Nicotine Withdrawal Symptoms in Animals Dysphoric?

As we have seen, a variety of behaviors are altered during nicotine withdrawal in rats. The question is whether these changes are dysphoric for the animals. This question has been largely ignored in the nicotine research literature, but it is in fact a crucial one. The observation that some behavioral changes are associated with nicotine withdrawal does not imply that these changes have anything to do with continued nicotine administration. The withdrawal symptoms must be aversive, or dysphoric, to motivate further drug intake and lead to drug dependence. None of the studies we reviewed provided evidence that the effects of nicotine withdrawal in rats are dysphoric.

Two intracranial self-stimulation studies addressed this issue. One showed increased thresholds for intracranial self-stimulation[164] during nicotine abstinence, indicating that abstinence was aversive. The other[101] showed increased responding when electrical current was withheld, and a trend towards increased rates in rewarded responding, suggesting that withdrawal was rewarding. These contradictory results, together with the doubtful utility of ICSS for assessing reinforcing properties of drugs (see Chapter 7), preclude drawing any clear conclusion from these studies.

The conditioned taste aversion (CTA) paradigm, which is commonly used to evaluate the aversive effects of acute or repeated drug administration, has also been employed to examine the affective value of the abstinence syndrome in rats. CTA is a useful paradigm for ascertaining the presence of an abstinence syndrome, particularly for those drugs in which dysphoric withdrawal symptoms are not obvious in spontaneous behavior. Both CTA and conditioned place aversion (CPA) to morphine withdrawal were readily demonstrated in several recent studies[e.g.,442,443]. Results for alcohol were inconclusive, as the "hangover" in rats appears to be characterized by pronounced adipsia, which masks any intake reduction resulting from CTA[202].

Spontaneous withdrawal from chronic nicotine failed to produce CTA in either rats[675] or mice[676]. Precipitated withdrawal by injecting the nicotine antagonist mecamylamine following chronic nicotine administration did produce CTA in rats in two studies by Suzuki and colleagues (Suzuki et al.,

1996; Suzuki et al., 1997). However, the significance of this finding is unclear, as another study[435] found that mecamylamine produced CTA in rats that were never treated with nicotine. Moreover, in the same study, animals that had been treated chronically with nicotine (for four times as long as in the studies of Suzuki and colleagues) actually showed conditioned taste *preference* following mecamylamine. Thus, in this latter study, precipitated withdrawal from nicotine was apparently rewarding.

5.   NICOTINE WITHDRAWAL IN HUMANS

The dysphoric smoking withdrawal syndrome in humans is defined in the DSM-IV as comprising eight central effects[10]: depressed mood, insomnia, irritability (or frustration, or anger), anxiety, difficulty concentrating, restlessness, decreased heart rate, increased appetite or weight gain. Other sources include also sadness and impatience[e.g.,145,326]. Apart from reduced heart rate and increased appetite, these symptoms are not specific to nicotine withdrawal, and may follow the interruption of a wide variety of normal and abnormal behavioral routines in which drug self-administration does not play a role[e.g.,10,403] (see Chapter 2). The only two abstinence symptoms that are nicotine-specific are reduced heart rate and increase in body weight[294]. Neither symptom is inherently dysphoric. Although weight gain is sometimes mentioned as a reason not to stop smoking, reluctance to gain weight is undoubtedly dependent on cultural values and individual variables.

5.1   Reversal of Smoking Withdrawal Symptoms

The cessation of heroin after chronic administration is followed by specific withdrawal symptoms that are fully reversed by re-administering heroin or other opiates. This observation underlies both the rationale for methadone maintenance programs for heroin-dependent individuals[62] and for "nicotine-replacement" treatment with nicotine gum and patches (see also Chapters 11 and 12). How effective is nicotine in reversing subjective withdrawal symptoms after smoking cessation?

According to a recent meta-analysis[654], "*nicotine replacement therapy reduces the severity of withdrawal symptoms in smokers abstaining from tobacco* (p. 1067)." Results from dozens of research reports support this conclusion. Many of these studies found that nicotine gum[e.g.,145,239,580], nasal nicotine spray[641], and especially transdermal nicotine patches[e.g.,2,130,132,659] [96,174,326,383,524,617] reduced some withdrawal symptoms. In *none* of these studies, however, did nicotine replacement abolish all withdrawal symptoms. Moreover, only one of these groups reported dose-related suppression of withdrawal symptoms[130], whereas several other studies[e.g.,237,258,373,699] found no relationship between nicotine dose and suppression of withdrawal symptoms. In fact, the last two studies[237,373], as well as a third one[492], did not find any effect of nicotine replacement on some, or all, of the subjective withdrawal symptoms.

There are two explanations that could account for the consistent observation that "nicotine replacement" devices suppress withdrawal only partially. The first is that not enough nicotine was provided. This is unlikely. Nicotine patches deliver sufficient nicotine to produce nausea in up to 40 percent of smokers, and still fail to abolish all withdrawal symptoms[327]. Moreover, even *ad libitum* self-administration of nicotine gum[e.g.,239] or 30 pieces of 2 mg gum[237] failed to provide full relief of withdrawal symptoms. Finally, as mentioned above, there is only a weak relationship, if at all, between the dose of nicotine and the degree of suppression of withdrawal symptoms[e.g.,237,258,373,699].

The second explanation might be that nicotine replacement does not mimic the rapid nicotine absorption in the bloodstream that characterizes tobacco smoking. This hypothesis is not plausible on theoretical grounds. If the smoker has blood levels of nicotine that are similar to those achieved by smoking, the presence of nicotine in the bloodstream should prevent withdrawal symptoms. How fast nicotine enters the blood stream may affect the pleasure the smoker derives, but not the withdrawal symptoms. Drug-specific withdrawal symptoms do not occur as long as a sufficiently high level of the drug is present in the brain – this is the reason that methadone can prevent opiate withdrawal symptoms for long duration even with slow delivery (oral intake)[311,358]. The hypothesis is also implausible on empirical grounds, as discussed in Chapter 8. Even a fast nicotine replacement (nasal spray) resulted only in partial suppression of withdrawal symptoms[641].

5.2   Dissociation of Subjective and Nicotine-Specific Withdrawal Symptoms

The discussion above suggests that the subjective withdrawal symptoms following smoking cessation may not depend on nicotine. This conclusion is strongly supported by direct empirical evidence. West and colleagues[699] had smokers switch from cigarettes containing, on the average, 1.3 mg of nicotine to ultra-light cigarettes containing 0.1 (less than 10 percent) mg of nicotine. Although this reduction in nicotine caused nicotine-specific withdrawal symptoms (increase in appetite and a reduction in heart rate), no subjective dysphoric withdrawal symptoms (irritability, depression, or inability to concentrate) were detected. In a more recent study[73], de-nicotinized cigarettes were found as effective as regular cigarettes in decreasing subjective withdrawal symptoms in 12-hour abstinent smokers, although they did not increase heart rate or plasma nicotine levels. These studies and others[e.g.,644] effectively demonstrate that the subjective withdrawal symptoms do not result from insufficient supply of nicotine.

Furthermore, if nicotine withdrawal were the cause of the subjective abstinence symptoms, withdrawal from nicotine replacement therapies should have produced the same symptoms. This is not the case: the symptoms produced by withdrawal from "nicotine replacement devices" are much weaker than those found in abstinent smokers[257,258].

Persuasive evidence against the hypothesis that subjective withdrawal symptoms are due to nicotine abstinence comes from work with the nicotine antagonist mecamylamine. When heroin addicts are injected with an opiate antagonist, an immediate and severe precipitated withdrawal syndrome follows[311]. In the same vein, mecamylamine should produce a precipitated withdrawal syndrome in smokers, similar to but more prompt than that following smoking cessation. As mentioned earlier, it does not[162,446,493,500,536,537]. Several studies reported that more cigarettes were smoked following mecamylamine[e.g.,446,536] but in no case was this increase significant compared to baseline rates. Moreover, none of these studies excluded the possibility that any change following mecamylamine could be due to its action on peripheral nicotine receptors involved in the subjective sensations provided by smoking.

Even more detrimental to the nicotine withdrawal hypothesis are the reports by Rose and his coworkers[536,537], that sustained mecamylamine pretreatment *reduces* smoking, as does nicotine. Furthermore, when nicotine and mecamylamine were administered together to smokers, they reduced smoking, smoking satisfaction, and craving more than either compound alone[536,537]. Thus, rather than opposing each other, as would be expected, the effects of the agonist and the antagonist were additive. These findings do not make sense pharmacologically. They can be easily explained, however, by considering that both nicotine and mecamylamine have side-effects that reduce smoking and are not mediated by the receptors for which they compete. One important side-effect could be nausea[649], as we discuss in greater detail in Chapter 12.

5.3   The Case of Ulcerative Colitis

A compelling way to demonstrate that nicotine causes physical dependence would be to conduct the following experiment. Eighty non-smokers, half never-smokers and half ex-smokers would be recruited. Half of each group would receive 15 mg of nicotine by transdermal patches for 16 hours a day for 12 weeks. This produces plasma levels of nicotine comparable to 35% of those of an average smoker[553]. The other half of the sample would receive placebo. At the end of 12 weeks the treatment would be discontinued and the participants forced to quit "cold turkey." If nicotine causes physical dependence, the never-smokers should experience craving for nicotine, expressed in subjective feelings of distress and perhaps in drug seeking behavior, such as continued purchase and use of transdermal patches. The ex-smokers, who have a certified history of long-term nicotine addiction, should feel even stronger cravings for nicotine, and a substantial proportion would be expected to relapse to smoking.

By sheer luck, this very experiment was indeed performed – not once, but as many times as nicotine was tested as a cure for the "non-smoker disease" called ulcerative colitis. The experiment described above[508] had as co-authors M.A.H. Russell and C. Feyerabend, two of the most productive researchers of nicotine addiction. This is how they summarize the results (under the title: *Mood Changes*, p. 814): *"During the trial most former smokers in the nicotine group felt well, but the life-long nonsmokers tolerated treatment with more difficulty. After the trial none reported a craving for smoking, and none reported any smoking during the subsequent 12 weeks.*"

Now let us conduct a 'thought experiment.' Imagine the same study, but this time with heroin instead of nicotine. In this experiment, heroin-naive and former heroin-dependent participants receive daily doses of heroin, providing approximately 35 percent of the dose consumed by an average heroin-dependent individual if he or she was allowed unlimited quantities (about 150 mg per day[564]) for 12 weeks. At the end of the 12 weeks, the participants are forced to quit 'cold turkey.' Is there anyone who believes that none of the participants will experience craving for heroin, and none, including the previously addicted participants, would self-administer heroin during the subsequent 12 weeks[H]?

Without claiming to be exhaustive, we found six more studies generally similar to that of Pullan et al.[231,241,560,652,653,670]. Incredibly, *none* of these studies reported withdrawal symptoms, renewed smoking in ex-smokers, or anything else that would suggest that patients became either addicted or re-addicted to nicotine. In our opinion, these results are nothing less than devastating for the nicotine addiction hypothesis. It is therefore remarkable that they are rarely cited in this context. The Citation Index lists 141 citations of the Pullan et al. article. Of these citations, 139 are confined to ulcerative colitis, and only two make any allusions to the implications for the smoking literature. We see this as a striking testimony to the reluctance of the scientific community to subject the nicotine addiction hypothesis to serious scrutiny.

6.   CONCLUSION

This chapter reviews the research pertaining to the accepted notion that animals and humans develop tolerance to and physical dependence on nicotine. There is no empirical evidence for tolerance to any reinforcing properties of nicotine (if such exist). In contrast to heroin and alcohol, humans do not increase their nicotine intake over time. Increased nicotine intake over time in animals has either not been reported, or was confounded

---

[H] With continuous 2 mg/kg/hour morphine release, osmotic minipumps turn naive rats into morphine addicts within 48 hours[399].

with increased nicotine-induced behavioral activation over time. The observations concerning physical dependence in rats, which are highly problematic by themselves, have not been replicated in humans. The smoking withdrawal syndrome in humans is entirely different from the nicotine abstinence syndrome in rats. It cannot be precipitated by opiate antagonists or, more importantly, by the nicotine antagonist mecamylamine. Moreover, it can be abolished by cigarettes that do not contain nicotine, whereas pure nicotine reduces it only partially. Finally, ex-smokers did not show any signs of craving nicotine after 12 weeks of exposure to nicotine at amounts comparable to 35% of the intake of an average smoker. We see the evidence presented in this chapter as adding up to a compelling case against the thesis that nicotine produces either tolerance to euphoric effects (if it has any) or dependence in humans.

Chapter 10

THE DIFFICULTY OF CURTAILING THE SMOKING HABIT

The notion that nicotine is as addictive as heroin has been explicitly voiced by government agencies such as the Surgeon General[665] and the Tobacco Advisory Group of The Royal College of Physicians[657]. Throughout this book, we have argued that this widely held notion is not supported by empirical evidence. As established in previous chapters (see also Chapter 13), the two compounds differ in their behavioral effects and in their positive and negative reinforcing properties both in animals and in humans. Whereas heroin consumption is associated with tolerance to the reinforcing effects and a dysphoric, drug-specific abstinence syndrome, neither syndrome can be established for nicotine, either in animals or in humans. As for compulsive use, in contrast to the opiate family, no evidence exists that humans voluntarily self-administer pure nicotine, be it in the form of transdermal patches, chewing gum, intranasal spray, or injection. Even when nicotine is used as an aid to smoking cessation, its administration (by supposedly nicotine-deprived humans) can best be described as compliance rather than as voluntary self-administration[e.g.,627, p. 35]. Similarly, there is no evidence of a single human non-smoker or ex-smoker having relapsed into, or even craved, pure nicotine after prolonged transdermal use[e.g.,508]. Based on our review so far, equating the addictive properties of nicotine and heroin appears to be more of a rhetorical exercise than an empirical statement.

A central argument marshaled by the Surgeon General and others[657,665] to justify the equation between heroin and nicotine has to do with the difficulty of quitting. Here is how the Surgeon General[665] (page 311) formulates this assertion: *"For many drug-dependent persons, achieving at least brief periods of drug abstinence is a readily achievable goal. Maintaining abstinence, or avoiding relapse, however, poses a much greater overall challenge."* After showing the strikingly similar one-year relapse curves for alcohol, heroin, and smoking abstinence, he states that *"... data from studies of alcohol, opioid, and tobacco relapse consistently support the similarities in relapse rates and patterns across these three forms of drug dependence, as well as the operation of similar determinants of relapse."* The implicit argument in this assertion is that if it is equally difficult to stop consuming heroin, alcohol, and nicotine, then these substances must be equally addictive. As we shall argue in this chapter, however, neither the premise nor its implicit consequence is valid.

First, we will show that the claim that the relapse rates of smoking and heroin use are similar is factually incorrect. The Surgeon General based his conclusion only on prospective studies with a maximum follow-up of one year. To remedy this omission, we shall expand the comparison of relapse rates to other indices of smoking abstinence. Our primary source will be retrospective studies, including some that are summarized by the Surgeon General himself.

Next, we will illustrate that quitting and relapse rates are not only a function of the chemical properties of a substance, but also strongly influenced by social pressures, legal status, availability, and beliefs. Thus, when comparing the quit rates of cigarettes and heroin, one must bear in mind that whereas heroin is illegal and therefore expensive, and obtaining it may be difficult if not dangerous, cigarettes are legal, affordable and widely available. As we show below, when these factors are considered, quitting smoking appears to be an entirely different endeavor from quitting habitual heroin use.

Finally, we will contend that even if one assumes that relapse rates of smoking are similar to those of heroin, it is erroneous to conclude that nicotine must be as addictive as heroin. This conclusion not only equates smoking with nicotine, it also disregards the fact that habits that do not involve drug consumption are often as difficult to break as heroin consumption. Therefore, the difficulty of quitting has no evidential weight for the question of nicotine's role in smoking. We have discussed this point earlier (see Chapter 2), and we shall re-address it here by comparing the success and relapse rates involved in smoking cessation and in dieting.

1. COMPLIANCE WITH LEGAL RESTRICTIONS

According to the Surgeon General, "*The pharmacologic and behavioral processes that determine tobacco addiction are similar to those that determine addiction to drugs such as heroin* ...(p. 9)[665]," and relapse rates for both "addictions" are the same. One way to examine this statement is to compare the effectiveness of the legal restrictions imposed on these habits.

A general characteristic of many psychoactive drugs (e.g., morphine, cocaine, and cannabis) is that the laws of most countries presently forbid their use. This was not always the case. During the 19th century laws did not regulate the use of opiates. Only in 1914, the USA set the modern precedent of outlawing morphine and heroin by passing the Harrison Act. From then on, the treatment of heroin addicts in the USA became mainly the task of the police, the law courts, and the penal system. Most countries in the Western World followed suit. Physicians were forbidden in most countries to prescribe opiates to addicts, who were expected to comply with the law and stop taking drugs. As the Surgeon General[665] aptly stated, however, "*drug-seeking and drug-taking behavior is driven by strong, often irresistible urges* (pp. 7–8)." Not surprisingly, these irresistible urges drive addicted individuals to break the law and, consequently, laws have not been very effective in controlling drug addiction.

The effectiveness of outlawing heroin was evaluated extensively by Brecher[62]. "*The only conclusion possible from either the FBND* [Federal Bureau of Narcotics and Dangerous Drugs] *or the NIMH* [National Institute of Mental Health] *is that the decades of enforcement of the Harrison Act and of countless other state and federal laws designed to stamp out opiate addiction have been a losing battle. There were almost certainly more opiate addicts in the United States from 1969 to 1971 than in 1914. And their status, of course, was far worse* (p. 62)." US government estimates of the number of heroin addicts in the USA ranged between 215,000 and 246,000 in 1914[62]. Current estimates range from 500,000 to 1,000,000 [88,251]. In the same time period, the US population increased from about 100 million to 272 million. Thus, the number of heroin addicts increased between 1914 and 1998 at least at the same rate as that of the population growth, demonstrating that the battle against heroin addiction in America has indeed been a losing one.

In contrast to the case of addictive drugs such as heroin, widespread legal restrictions on smoking in the Western Hemisphere are quite recent. When the authors of this book were students, both professors and students in Israel were allowed to smoke during lectures, and they often did. In fact, with the exclusion of gas stations and other places in which smoking could be disastrous, smoking was permitted pretty much everywhere. Bed-ridden patients in hospitals were allowed to smoke even when other patients shared the same room. Movie theaters were dense with smoke, as were buses, trains, and elevators. Non-smoking seats in airplanes were rare, and smokeless flights were unheard of. All of this has changed, and in contrast to the case of heroin, compliance with smoking restrictions, in Israel and around the world, has been remarkable. During the 18 years that have passed since No Smoking signs were installed at Tel Aviv University, we have never seen, or even heard of, a single transgression in our classes. The Israeli student apparently finds it easier to refrain from smoking in the classroom than to overcome other irresistible urges, like being late or talking to his or her neighbor during lectures.

Smoking restrictions have reduced smoking overall, not only in those places in which smoking was expressly forbidden. Recent studies of the effects of restricted smoking in the work place[e.g.,63,64,67,290,319,466] found that restrictions significantly decreased overall smoking (measured by the number of cigarettes), in some cases by 25 percent or more[91,172,724]. Thus, smokers apparently do not compensate substantially for these restrictions by smoking more when they leave the work place. Some studies[e.g.,171,210,466] show that restrictions may even facilitate complete smoking cessation. Similar effects were also reported with household restrictions on smoking[53].

Thus, in contrast to the laws forbidding heroin use, restrictions on smoking are effective. However, this may not be a fair comparison, as smoking restrictions are limited to certain times and places while the ban on heroin use is total. We have no way of knowing how many smokers would quit if, like heroin, tobacco products would be outlawed entirely. Yet, the studies cited above show that smokers generally will comply with restrictions and reduce their smoking quite readily under these circumstances. Moreover, the majority of smokers not only comply with smoking restrictions in the work place but actually favor such restrictions[e.g.,14,63,421].

2. MEASURING THE DIFFICULTY OF ABSTINENCE: PROSPECTIVE AND RETROSPECTIVE METHODS

There are two main methods of assessing the difficulty of breaking unwanted habits, whether or not these habits involve drugs. The first method is the prospective study, generally aimed at testing a method for abstaining from a given 'bad habit' (overeating, nail biting, heroin use, smoking, etc.). In a typical treatment study participants, who are either recruited or self-referred, are assigned to a treatment procedure, a 'placebo' treatment or a wait-list control group. In studies that examine self-quitting, no treatment is given. Abstinence or relapse is measured after a certain time period, which tends to be highly variable across studies. A low degree of abstinence, or a high rate of relapse, is taken to reflect the difficulty of kicking the habit under study.

The second method of measuring the difficulty of quitting is the retrospective study. In its simplest form, a retrospective study quantifies the percentage of a sample[566] or a population[665] that currently abstains from unwanted behavior practiced in the past. If a large percentage has abstained from habit X, whereas a small percentage has abstained from habit Y, it can be inferred that, all other things being equal, it is easier to quit X than Y. As we shall see, prospective and retrospective studies often yield widely diverging estimates of the difficulty of quitting smoking.

2.1 Prospective studies: limited-time smoking cessation rates

How hard is it for smokers to stop smoking for limited periods? The Jewish religion forbids smoking on the Sabbath for approximately 24 hours, and even hard-core smokers are able to comply with this rule on a weekly basis. But what about longer periods, say several weeks or months? An obvious place to look for answers is in the results of prospective studies investigating smoking cessation following treatment. Unfortunately, there are hundreds, possibly thousands, of reports on smoking cessation trials, which vary in subject selection, treatment procedure, duration of treatment and follow-up, choice of control groups or placebo, methods of verifying cessation, etc.

One way to reduce the confusion is to appeal to statistical summaries of smoking cessation studies. There exist numerous meta-analyses of specific treatment methods[e.g.,36,89,175,608], and one mega-meta-analysis comprising 633 studies of smoking cessation methods of varying types[587]. However, as the focus of the treatment studies is on complete smoking cessation, generally defined as one-year complete abstinence, information on shorter cessation intervals is often missing. In addition, several of these meta-analyses report only odds ratios, which basically express how much more effective a given treatment is compared to placebo or control groups. Although this information is valid and meaningful in deciding whether a treatment is better than its control, it does not allow determination of cessation rates. Furthermore, specific data on quitting rates of participants in control groups or groups receiving placebo treatment are often lacking. These data would constitute a meaningful estimate of unaided quitting, an issue we shall address later in this chapter.

Schwartz[587] summarized follow-up outcomes of smoking cessation trials conducted between 1959 and 1985. Depending on the kind of treatment, a 33 percent rate of abstinence for 6 months was reported in up to 89 percent of the studies. These figures, however, may not accurately reflect the current state of affairs. The primary reason for this caveat is that only a few of the studies reviewed by Schwartz were nicotine replacement studies, as these were just beginning to gain in popularity when Schwartz's review was conducted[587]. Therefore, we examined recent meta-analyses of nicotine replacement studies to supplement these data.

Several meta-analyses were conducted to determine the effectiveness of nicotine replacement for quitting smoking (see Chapter 11). However, most of these investigations reported only one-year cessation rates. An exception is a 1993 meta-analysis[89] of 33 studies that examined the effectiveness of nicotine gum. According to this analysis, short-term cessation (up to 8 weeks) was obtained by about 55–70 percent of the participants, if the gum was an adjunct to a minimum of 3 hours of intensive therapy. Without such therapy, about 38–42 percent of the participants achieved short-term cessation. Intensive therapy with placebo gum, and with no gum at all, resulted in short-term cessation rates of about 50 and 40 percent, respectively. In a brief treatment condition, these figures were about 32 and 20 percent. Another meta-analysis of 17 trials of transdermal patches worn for 4–8 weeks[176] found overall abstinence rates of 27 percent for the active patch and 13 percent for placebo patches at the end of treatment. These figures were down to 22 and 9 percent, respectively, at the 6-months follow-up point.

Because of the large variability of the data from the various reviews, it is impossible to conclude how difficult short-term cessation is for untreated (control and placebo) participants. Regarding treated participants, however, the recent figures do not invalidate Schwartz's estimates. We may conclude that nearly one third of smokers who received active treatment achieved short-term (up to 6 months) cessation[587]. It is reasonable to assume that a greater proportion of participants can stop smoking for shorter periods, but present data do not allow us to estimate this proportion reliably.

2.2   Prospective studies: Complete cessation rates

Just as prospective smoking cessation studies vary tremendously in reported rates of short-term cessation, they also vary in obtained rates of quitting, defined in this literature as one year of complete abstinence. On the basis of the 1987 meta-analysis conducted by Schwartz[587] (see above), Viswesvaran and Schmidt[677] compared the effectiveness of various smoking cessation methods. The results, not always tested after one year, were strikingly heterogeneous. The lowest quitting rate was obtained following physician's advice (17 studies, 7 percent success rate). Most behaviorally oriented programs did quite well: hypnosis (48 studies, 36% success), smoke aversion (103 studies, 31% success), group withdrawal (46 studies, 30% success) and even acupuncture (19 studies, 30% success) were effective in close to one third of the participants. Notably, the pharmacologically oriented programs were far less effective. Nicotine chewing gum (40 studies, 16% success) and medication-based programs (29 studies, 18% success) did only half as well as psychological treatment. However, alternative nicotine replacement methods, including nicotine patches, inhalers, nasal spray, and sublingual tablets were not available at the time. We shall review newer studies that examined the (still modest) success of these devices in Chapter 11.

Not surprisingly, highly motivated participants such as pulmonary patients (17 studies, 34% success) and cardiac patients (34 studies, 42% success) were the most successful quitters. We shall expand on this finding later, in discussing the role of motivation for quitting. Finally, according to Viswesvaran and Schmidt's calculations[677], "*on average, only 6.4 percent of the smokers could be expected to quit smoking without any intervention* (p. 554)."

3.   COMPLETE CESSATION IN RETROSPECTIVE STUDIES

The results of prospective studies, presented above, lead to the conclusion that whereas a brief abstinence of hours and days does not seem to present a problem for most smokers, abstinence for more substantial periods is achieved by only a minority of smokers. Findings obtained by retrospective studies, however, seem to paint an entirely different picture. Below, we review the reality of smoking cessation according to retrospective studies, and attempt to reconcile it with the reality gleaned from the prospective approach.

In a controversial 1982 study[566], the prominent social psychologist Stanley Schachter interviewed the entire staff of a psychology department including academic staff, technicians, secretaries, and graduate students and a large portion of the working population of a small town. He asked the participants whether they had smoked, whether they had attempted to quit and whether they had succeeded in doing so. Schachter found that 63.6 percent of the smokers who attempted to quit had succeeded, and that the vast majority of successful quitters overcame the habit without professional assistance. Using a similar methodology, Rzewnicki and Forgays[557] interviewed all those having a mailbox in the Psychology Department of the University of Vermont and reported a successful quitting ratio of 50 percent. This group also replicated Schachter's observation that most quitters ceased smoking unassisted.

These results are puzzling, to say the least, in light of the figures provided by prospective studies and the Surgeon General's[665] claim that smoking cessation rates are as low as those obtained with heroin. They are especially puzzling considering the fact that the majority of Schachter's interviewees had quit without help. One solution to the apparent incongruity is to discard the retrospective figures as anomalies, as Viswesvaran and Schmidt[677] apparently did when they stated that only 6.4 percent of smokers could be expected to quit smoking without any intervention. As will presently become evident, however, the findings of the retrospective studies are no anomalies; in fact, they are corroborated by very reliable sources, including the Surgeon General himself.

According to the Surgeon General's report[665], millions of Americans, Canadians, and British have stopped smoking over the years. Since 1965, when 52.1 percent of American adult males smoked, the percentage of adult male smokers declined to 34.8 percent in 1983 and to 32.7 percent in 1986. This decrease, of approximately one percent per year, is nearly linear in most of the populations in the Surgeon General's survey[665]. More recent figures indicate that the percentage of adult smokers has continued to decline from 1988 to 24.7 percent in 1997[425], at a little slower rate than during the two decades before. Thus, the prevalence of smoking has declined by over 50 percent in three decades.

Not all of this decrease in the number of smokers is attributable to quitting. Prevention of smoking, especially at younger ages, could well be another prominent factor[665]. However, the Surgeon General[665] also reported directly measured estimates of quitting. In 1985, the quit ratio (proportion of former smokers in a given population divided by the proportion of that population who had ever been smokers) reached 33 percent in males aged 25–34, 45 percent in males aged 35–44, 55 percent in males aged 45–64, and a whopping 70 percent in males over 65 years of age. These figures are not discrepant from those reported in the two retrospective studies described above[557,566].

As the data presented above are tabulated by age, they do not allow an estimation of the quitting ratio for the entire population. Surveys in Great Britain, however, did report the overall population smoking cessation rate, and it is a very substantial one: Over the last 25 years, about 50% percent of smokers have stopped smoking before the age of 60[657]. Given that at least 42 percent of British smokers declare that they do not want to quit[452] and assuming that this proportion remains stable over time, it follows that a majority of (British) smokers who want to quit can eventually achieve this goal.

Related estimates were also reported for the USA population. The Surgeon General[665] stated (p. 565): "*Based on population estimates and the NHIS* [National Health Interview Surveys], *the total number of adult smokers (aged 20 years and older) in the United States declined from approximately 52,400,000 in 1976 to approximately 51,100,000 in 1985. The total number of former smokers increased from approximately 29,500,000 to 40,900,000 within this time period.*" Thus, over 11 million Americans quit smoking in the period of one decade, compared to approximately 10 millions who joined the ranks of smokers during the same period. In fact, as smoking prevalence in the adult population decreased by 6.3 percent between 1976 and 1985[665] and by another 5.7 percent until 1997[425], the number of former smokers in the USA should presently be higher than the number of smokers. In light of these trends, the high rates of quitters reported by the two retrospective studies cited above[557,566] no longer appear to be an anomaly.

4.   SINGLE-TRIAL *VS.* MULTI-TRIAL CESSATION RATES

As we showed above, prospective studies paint a rather pessimistic picture of smokers' ability to kick their habit, whereas retrospective surveys show that most smokers who attempt to quit eventually succeed. For reasons we consider in Chapter 13, the pessimistic picture is the one that has been dominant in the research literature, and even more so in government publications and the media. The Surgeon General, for one, largely ignored the implications of retrospective studies, including data provided in his own report, when he claimed that quitting smoking is as difficult as quitting heroin. In order to reach a rational and objective picture of the difficulty of quitting smoking, it is essential to understand and resolve the discrepancy between prospective and retrospective data. The key for resolving this contradiction, as others have noted[e.g.,108], is to understand the difference between single-trial and multi-trial cessation rates.

The statistics provided by the Surgeon General (e.g., that 70 percent of male smokers over 65 years of age had quit) and by the two retrospective studies discussed above (e.g., that 63.6 percent of the smokers in Schachter's study had quit) do not reveal what the *single-trial* quitting odds are or how many trials smokers need to stop permanently. Conversely, the cumulative *multi-trial* chance of success cannot be inferred from the probability of success in a single unassisted trial. To determine this cumulative rate we need to know (a) the single-trial success rate, (b) how many trials motivated smokers are willing to make, and (c) whether and how chances of success per trial change with repeated trials.

Cohen et al.[108] supplied part of this information. On the basis of ten independent studies, these authors showed that first-time self-quitters have the same chance of success as those who have tried 6 times or more. They also cited an unpublished study[114] showing that in people who made up to 9 attempts, success-rates and number of cessation attempts are not related. The implication of these statistics is that a smoker's chance of succeeding in any given cessation attempt does not depend on how many previous attempts he or she had made. Indeed, many smokers go through numerous quitting attempts before finally succeeding. One study, for example[374] reported that 14.9 percent of the participants in one treatment condition had attempted to quit 10 times or more[1].

Figure 1 illustrates how successive attempts, each with a fixed probability of success, can result in the population cessation rates reported by retrospective studies. With each attempt, the remaining population of smokers is reduced by a fixed percentage, equal to the single-trial success rate. One curve represents a low single-trial success rate of 5 percent, which is the median of the 10 prospective studies reported by Cohen et al. (1989). With this rate, the number of attempts required to reach the 33 percent quit

---

[1] We would like to remark that these observations contradict hypotheses postulating that some smokers remain addicted because of personality or genetic factors. These hypotheses imply that self-quitting may be quite feasible for individuals who are not predisposed to smoking addiction but harder, or impossible, for those who are. If this were the case, individuals with the genetic or personality disposition to nicotine addiction would constitute an increasingly higher percentage of unsuccessful self-quitters. This should lead to a cumulative reduction in success-rate over repeated quitting trials. That this does not happen[108,114] suggests that success in quitting depends on other factors, perhaps primarily on motivation (see discussion at the end of this chapter).

ratio reported for 25–34 year-old men and women[665] is 8, which is well within the range of quitting attempts made by smokers[108,114,374]. If we assume a single-trial success-rate of 14 percent – the lowest of the success rates in the Finnish study, and the highest of the Cohen studies – the number of attempts necessary to reach 33 percent is only 3 (see Figure 1). In order to attain the higher quit ratios reported by Schachter[566] and Rzewnicki and Forgays[557], 4–6 trials would be needed.

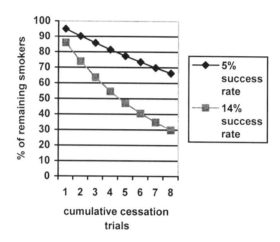

Figure 10.1. Cumulative effect of repeated cessation attempts with a 5 or 14% success rate on a smoking population

The percentage of abstinent smokers in the general population who are assisted by professionals is not known, and may well be as low as Schachter found. Smoking cessation treatments are typically costly, and it is unlikely that a large proportion of those who attempt to quit several times do so by using professional help repeatedly. However, if the success rate of treatments, relative to self-quitting, is high, it would account for any remaining gap between the observed proportion of ex-smokers in the population[557,566,665] and the rate reported in prospective single-trial studies in self-quitters[635].

5. SUMMARY: THE SIMILARITY OF SMOKING AND HEROIN ABSTINENCE RATES

The Surgeon General, whom we cited at the beginning of this chapter, showed that the one-year abstinence rates for heroin and smoking are very similar. He went on to infer that (1) smoking is as difficult to quit as heroin and alcohol, and that, therefore, (2) nicotine is as addictive as alcohol and heroin. We are now in the position to evaluate the validity of the first inference. We will proceed to discuss the second in the next section.

As we have seen, the picture painted by prospective studies of smoking cessation is entirely different from the one painted by retrospective ones. In supporting his statement that it is as difficult to quit smoking as it is to quit heroin, the Surgeon General relied only on prospective studies. Had he included retrospective data as well, this dramatic statement would not be defensible. Specifically, we have shown that the percentage of heroin addicts in the general population has remained relatively constant over 8 decades, whereas the proportional percentage of smokers decreased by over 50 percent in 35 years. One explanation for this difference is that once smokers quit for a year, they are likely to remain abstinent, whereas heroin addicts are likely to relapse to drug use even after prolonged abstinence. Thus, although relapse rates following heroin abstinence and smoking cessation are the same at the one-year mark, as the Surgeon General stated, the multi-trial or cumulative relapse rates may be entirely different.

6. OVEREATING: ANOTHER IRRESISTIBLE URGE

We have shown above that despite the Surgeon General's claims, the long-term relapse rates for heroin and smoking are quite different. Even if they were the same, however, this would constitute absolutely no support for the claim that nicotine is addictive. As we have shown in our discussion of compulsive habits, many non-chemical habits are as difficult to quit as the most addictive drugs. The Surgeon General failed to include such non-chemical habits in his comparison of relapse rates. This omission is unlikely to have been accidental. The Surgeon General wanted to draw from his relapse-rate comparison the inference that smoking is as addictive as heroin and alcohol. Had he included non-chemical habits in his comparison, this inference would have been instantly refuted.

We have argued earlier that relapse, just like craving, compulsive use, or fixed patterns of use, does not distinguish drug addiction from compulsive habits. In that context, we mentioned nail biting, pathological gambling, kleptomania, trichotillomania, sexual paraphillias and other compulsions that are characterized by high relapse rates. In this section, we intend to buttress this argument by exploring the relapse rates associated with overeating. We chose overeating because, like smoking and heroin addiction, it is a major health problem about which both prospective and retrospective data are available. If success and relapse rates for dieting are similar to the corresponding figures for smoking cessation, then clearly such data cannot be used to judge whether or not a habit is maintained by chemical addiction.

Obesity is a major health hazard, increasing the risk of serious medical problems such as type 2 diabetes, gallbladder disease and high blood pressure[439]. It has been estimated that the number of annual deaths of adults in the USA caused by obesity is about 325,000 amongst nonsmokers and never-smokers[9]. Obesity is an increasingly common problem. According to one estimate, one in two adults in the United States is overweight or obese[179] and a recent study[429] estimated that in specific populations, obesity has increased by up to 20 percent from 1991 to 1998. The increase in prevalence varied by region, ranging from a relatively small increase of 11.3 percent for Delaware to 101.8 percent for Georgia.

Obesity and smoking share the characteristics of high morbidity and mortality. It is therefore not surprising that many people try to lose weight for the same reason that many attempt to quit smoking. In surveys conducted between 1985 and 1988, 48 percent of the women and 29 percent of the men reported that they were trying to lose weight[591]. In similar surveys conducted between 1989 and 1992, these figures were 41 and 26 percent, respectively[591]. Methods included counting calories, participation in organized weight loss programs, using dietary supplements, taking diet pills, and fasting[592]. As in the case of smoking, prospective studies indicate that whereas short-term weight loss is quite feasible, significant long-term weight loss is a very difficult endeavor[e.g.,236,284]. Only 3 percent of the participants in weight loss programs achieve long-term weight loss[357] and complete relapse is the rule after 3–5 years[423].

There is one major difference between quitting smoking and dieting. Whereas the percentage of smokers in the US population is on the decline, having dropped to less than half what it was 35 years ago[425,665], the prevalence of obesity is on the increase. With over 40 percent of all American women and over 25 percent of all American men dieting, the lack of success in losing weight can hardly be attributed to lack of trying. It seems rather that it is easier to refrain from smoking after one has quit than to avoid regaining weight after one has succeeded in losing the excessive pounds. Thus, though quitting smoking may be difficult, dieting seems to be at least as difficult or even more difficult, despite the fact that overeating does not involve a psychoactive drug. Hence the purported similarity between the relapse rates of heroin, alcohol and nicotine tells us nothing about the extent to which nicotine is addictive or the role it may have in maintaining the smoking habit.

7. THE IMPORTANCE OF MOTIVATION FOR QUITTING

An oft-cited British survey[452] reported that 48 percent of smokers of all ages had not abstained from smoking for as long as a week during the past 5 years. This observation was interpreted by others[635] as evidence that a large proportion of smokers are *unable* to stop smoking for as long as a week. This interpretation ignores the fact that 42 percent of adult smokers in the same survey reported that they *did not want* to give up smoking altogether. It is likely, therefore, that the majority of smokers in this survey who reported that they had never abstained for more than a week were simply unwilling, rather than unable, to do so. It would probably be uncontested that the wish to give up smoking is a necessary condition for smoking cessation, whether on a permanent basis or for only a week. Below, we explore the role of motivation for smoking cessation.

7.1 The Independence of Declaration

The British survey cited above[452] reported that whereas 58 percent of the smokers wished to quit, only 13 percent thought that they would be likely to succeed were they to decide to give up smoking in the next 3 months. These statistics appear to indicate that most smokers have a high degree of motivation to quit smoking, which is tragically throttled by a sense of hopelessness about their ability to do so. It is essential to remember, however, that these results reflect smokers' self-reported attitudes and intentions, the validity of which has been questioned since the early days of social psychology. Studies have consistently shown that attitudes and behaviors are often only modestly correlated[367,453 207,222,223,642]. In the area of health behaviors, specifically, the correspondence between declaring and acting on the wish to relinquish bad habits and to adopt healthy and wholesome ones in their stead is often marginal[205,339,340,643].

The validity of such declarations has been questioned specifically with regard to smoking, an area in which respondents have many reasons to declare their wish and intention to quit. As Kozlowski and colleagues[355] asked: "*How better for a smoker to avoid the pesterings of a physician or other interviewer than to say (whether believing it or not) that he wants to and has even tried to give up cigarettes* (p. 699)?" We would add that admitting a lack of desire to stop smoking would make the responder appear – in others' eyes as well as in his or her own – not only irrational, but decidedly not politically correct. But what does such a declaration mean? Kozlowski et al.[355] described a survey in Philadelphia, where 4,775 out of 11,709 smoking respondents said they would be interested in stopping smoking if a smoking cessation clinic were set up. Only 257, however, attended a preliminary meeting about the clinic and once it was established, only 150 made use of it. There is good reason to doubt, therefore, that a survey-expressed wish to stop smoking is a valid indicator of either strong motivation or serious intention to do so.

7.2 The Role of Motivation in Cessation Studies

While it seems obvious that the success of cessation attempts depends on the smoker's motivation to quit, this issue is rarely addressed in cessation studies.   As mentioned earlier, participants in these studies are either self-referred or recruited. Self-referred participants are generally motivated by a wish to stop the bad habit in question.   In the case of recruited participants, it is often difficult to determine whether their motivation is boosted by external incentives such as money, or whether they enroll in the study when their motivation is at a peak.   There is considerable evidence that these factors may make a significant difference.   For example, in a meta-analysis of 6 transdermal patch studies of variable duration[648] the success rate of self-referred participants (8–16%) was significantly greater than that of participants who were invited to participate in the studies (2– 10%).

In most prospective studies, cessation trials commence when the investigator is ready to start the study, but not necessarily when the participants are at their peak of motivation.   Motivation to quit varies between smokers, and very likely also during the lifetime of every smoker. When coughing becomes daily, when asthma attacks and chest pains begin to be worrisome, motivation to quit may be significantly stronger than when smoking has no observable negative effects.   As mentioned earlier, highly motivated participants such as pulmonary and cardiac patients did best in a meta-analysis of smoking cessation studies[677].

The messy issues involved in subject recruiting can be gleaned from a study[293] where smokers *"that were about to quit on their own* (p. 689)" were recruited by radio and newspaper advertisements and offered payment for filling out forms. Participants were unaware of the amount of payment ($20) until after entering the study.   Clearly, the initial motivation of the participants to quit was confounded by, amongst other factors, the promise of an unknown sum of money.   Furthermore, out of 1,396 individuals who applied for the study, the author excluded 41 percent.   One of the criteria for exclusion was the author's judgment that the candidate had *"little motivation for cessation* (p. 689)."   It is unclear how this was determined, and it remains quite possible that some participants succeeded in "faking" motivation in order to be included.

The importance of motivation for successful quitting is especially evident in studies where all participants are self-selected. A recent Finnish report[351] tested the rate of abstinence following a "Quit and Win" contest. Participants in this study are likely to have been highly motivated as they were not only self-selected, but also driven by the competitive setting.   Without any treatment, between 46 and 50 percent of the participants abstained for a month (non-responders were counted as non-abstaining).   A follow-up reported 14–19 percent one-year abstinence rates, higher than the highest of Cohen et al.[108] studies.

8.   CONCLUSION

This chapter focused on the Surgeon General's assertion that smoking abstinence rates are similar to those found for heroin and alcohol and on the popularized inference from this assertion, namely that nicotine is as addictive as heroin and alcohol.   We argued that both the assertion and the ensuing deduction are false.   We began by showing that smokers have been remarkably compliant with smoking regulations, whereas outlawing heroin has entirely failed to affect heroin use.   We proceeded to show that the Surgeon General based his abstinence rate comparison only on prospective studies with a maximum follow-up of one year.   Once retrospective data are considered, smoking cessation appears to be much more feasible and commonplace than cessation of heroin.   We went on to argue that even if relapse rates of smoking were similar to those of heroin, the inference that nicotine is as addictive as heroin does not follow, either logically or empirically.   To recapitulate this point we compared the success and relapse rates associated with smoking cessation and with dieting.   This comparison underscored our claim that the difficulty of abstaining from unhealthy habits does not testify to the presence of psychoactive drugs.   Finally, we explored the role of motivation, a factor that is often disregarded or downplayed in smoking cessation research.

Chapter 11

"NICOTINE REPLACEMENT THERAPIES"

Two assumptions motivated the development and testing of so-called nicotine replacement therapies[657](NRTs). The first was that nicotine is addictive in much the same way that heroin is[665] and the second, that nicotine is the major cause of cigarette smoking. Just as methadone helps heroin-dependent individuals break their addiction, providing nicotine to smokers via a route other than smoking was expected to minimize withdrawal symptoms, craving and relapse. *"The basic idea behind using nicotine replacement is to break the quitting process into two phases. In the first phase, smokers learn to cope without smoking behaviour and regular rapid boli of nicotine, while protected from the worst withdrawal effects by moderate levels of nicotine provided by NRT. Later, nicotine is gradually withdrawn completely* (p.143)[657].*"* Nicotine gum, transdermal patches, nicotine spray, nicotine inhalers, and nicotine sublingual tablets were produced according to this rationale, and their effectiveness is commonly cited as the ultimate evidence for the nicotine addiction hypothesis. In discussing this book with colleagues, we have often encountered variations of the following question: *"If you claim that nicotine is not addictive, how come nicotine gum and patches are so effective for quitting?"*

We will begin this short chapter by examining the purported success of "nicotine replacement" treatments for smoking cessation, and show that the efficacy of nicotine gum and patches is actually very modest. We will then compare these treatments to methadone treatment for opiate addiction, in order to demonstrate that their effects and, very likely, their mechanisms of action, are entirely different. Finally, we will offer several alternative explanations for the facilitative effect of "nicotine replacement" devices for smoking cessation. These alternative explanations, which have nothing to do with "replacement," demonstrate that the success of NRTs has no bearing on the nicotine addiction hypothesis.

1.   THE LIMITED EFFICACY OF "NICOTINE REPLACEMENT" DEVICES

Nicotine chewing gum, the first of the NRT devices, is available in 2 and 4 mg doses. Its recommended use is to chew each piece slowly for 30 minutes and to use up to 15 pieces per day. At the highest dose, about 1.2 mg of nicotine reaches the bloodstream. Nicotine sublingual tablets, a similar device, are held under the tongue until they dissolve. The dose delivered by these tablets is similar to that of the nicotine gum.

Nicotine transdermal patches can deliver up to approximately 1 mg of nicotine per hour, either around the clock or for 16 hours per day. In contrast to nicotine chewing gum and sublingual tablets, both of which cause nicotine blood levels to reach a plateau after about 30 minutes, it takes hours for such levels to be reached with transdermal patches.

The device that offers the most rapid delivery amongst the NRTs is the nicotine nasal spray. Blood levels of nicotine reach a plateau after about 10 minutes. A single spray of the nicotine solution delivers about 0.5 mg of nicotine. In spite of this rapid delivery, there is no evidence that this nicotine replacement device is more efficacious than any of the others[246], which is clearly at odds with the popular delivery kinetics hypothesis (see Chapter 8).

The nicotine inhaler is a plastic device resembling a cigarette that contains a cartridge with a polythene nicotine-impregnated plug[657]. The user is advised to puff on the inhaler intensively and frequently, as the amount of nicotine absorbed with the inhaler is very small: twenty puffs on the inhaler provide about the same amount of nicotine as one puff on a cigarette.

Several meta-analyses have examined the efficacy of nicotine replacement devices, mainly nicotine gum and transdermal patches, for smoking cessation. On the basis of the 1987 meta-analysis conducted by

Schwartz[587], Viswesvaran and Schmidt[677] (see also previous chapter) compared the effectiveness of various smoking cessation methods. Among other methods, they examined the efficacy of nicotine gum, the only NRT available at the time Schwartz collected his data. The overall complete cessation rate for smokers using nicotine gum, based on 40 studies, was 16 percent. This rate is rather unimpressive, especially considering that many of these studies examined cessation rates for relatively short periods.

A 1993 meta-analysis[89] summarizing 33 studies of nicotine gum treatment reported that a short-term cessation (up to 8 weeks) rate was achieved by 55–70 percent of the participants. However, this rate was obtained when the gum was used as an adjunct to a minimum of 3-hour group or individual psychotherapy ("intensive treatment"). When nicotine gum was used without psychotherapy ("brief treatment"), about 38–42 percent of the participants achieved short-term cessation. Moreover, psychotherapy alone was as effective as the nicotine gum, resulting in a short-term cessation rate of 40 percent. When placebo gum was added to the psychotherapy, 50 percent of the participants achieved short-term cessation, exceeding the efficacy of the nicotine gum. Finally, when placebo gum was used with the "brief treatment," short-term cessation was achieved by 32 percent of smokers. Thus, in this meta-analysis, nicotine gum exceeded placebo gum only by 6–10 percent.

Although the transdermal nicotine patch appears to be *"one of the most popular cessation methods used by smokers* (p. S63)[124]*,"* its actual effectiveness is not impressive. A meta-analysis of 17 studies in which patches were used for 4–18 weeks[176] reported overall abstinence rates of 27 percent for the active patch and 13 percent for the placebo patch at the end of treatment. After 6 months, these figures were 22 and 9 percent, respectively. At this point, then, nicotine patches exceeded placebo patches by 13 percent, but their overall efficacy was still unimpressive.

The long-term efficacy of transdermal patches is even more disappointing. One meta-analysis of studies testing the effectiveness of nicotine patches reported an overall one-year abstinence rate of only 9 percent[648]. Another meta-analysis[523] reported that the range of one-year abstinence rates was between 9 and 28 percent. In the largest study reviewed in this meta-analysis, which included nearly as many participants as all other studies combined, the nicotine patch resulted in only 11 percent success, compared to 8 percent success with a placebo patch! Notably, the most successful studies in this meta-analysis did not rely on patches alone, but provided extensive support and advice during treatment.

Finally, a meta-analysis[608] combining 42 gum studies (30 followed up for one year, 12 for six months) and 9 patch studies (followed up for a year) reported that 19 percent of the participants on NRT quit smoking, compared to 11 percent of the participants in control groups. Thus, the mean gain in cessation rate attributable to "nicotine replacement" devices was 8 percent.

2.   METHADONE TREATMENT FOR OPIATE ADDICTION

The tremendous difficulty involved in withdrawal from opiate addiction stimulated Dole and Nyswander, joined later by Kreek, to search for a way to help addicts refrain from self-administering heroin. Their solution, established in the sixties, became known as "long-term methadone maintenance treatment[358]." Their pioneering methods were implemented in many countries and methadone treatment has provided a way back to society for countless heroin addicts. The treatment consists of "... *administering it* [methadone] *by the oral route in one dose each day. After initial stabilization on 20–40 mg/day, which prevented withdrawal signs and symptoms, the dose was slowly escalated (at a rate we now recommend not to exceed 10 mg/week) up to a full treatment dose of usually 80–120 mg/day. Once patients were stabilized on such a dose, there were no narcotic-like effects and no symptoms of narcotic withdrawal, and we found that "drug hunger" or craving had also abated and then disappeared in most patients* (p. 558)[358]."

Methadone acts on the same receptors as heroin; consequently, it will block the action of superimposed heroin. "*In each case, the addict, achieving no euphoric effects from superimposed self-administered illicit heroin, has to make an important decision: whether to stop methadone treatment to be able to get the "high" or euphoric effects from heroin, or to accept the stabilizing effects of methadone maintenance treatment, with its prevention of opiate withdrawal and reduction or elimination of drug craving. Numerous studies have shown that the majority of patients in early treatment will conduct such self-experimentation during the first 3–6 months of treatment and then will elect to stay in methadone maintenance treatment* (p. 559)[358]."

3.   METHADONE MAINTENANCE VS. "NICOTINE REPLACEMENT" THERAPY

There are essential differences between methadone maintenance and nicotine "replacement" therapies that somehow escaped the full attention of the Surgeon General and of most smoking researchers. We shall review these differences here with the intent of showing that, contrary to common wisdom, the two types of treatment have very little in common.

Firstly, although methadone may not bring about complete opiate detoxification[150], it is extremely effective in stopping participants from self-administering heroin for long periods of time[358,637]. In contrast, as we have seen above, the efficacy of nicotine gum and patches in producing smoking cessation rarely exceeds 11–15 percent of the smokers, which is lower than most non-"replacement" treatments. This observation clearly contradicts the nicotine addiction hypothesis, which predicts that as smoking essentially means self-administering nicotine, smokers should stop smoking if supplied with nicotine by other routes.

Secondly, as methadone acts on the same receptors as do heroin and morphine, it has the same potential as do the other opiates (depending on the route of administration) for producing physical dependence, tolerance and abstinence symptoms in drug-naive individuals. In contrast, non-smokers do not use nicotine gum or patches voluntarily, and certainly do not become addicted to them[292]. As we have seen, Pullan et al.[508] demonstrated that 12 weeks of treatment by transdermal nicotine patches did not re-addict ex-smokers: not a single one expressed even a craving for cigarettes after being exposed to levels of nicotine comparable to 35% of those delivered by daily cigarettes of the average smoker for 12 weeks. It has been reported that some ex-smokers use nicotine gum for long periods after smoking cessation [54,245,257,298]. This continued use, however, demonstrates that smokers *believe* that the gum facilitates quitting, not that the gum actually provides smokers with their drug of dependence.

Finally, methadone fully suppresses the withdrawal symptoms caused by abstinence from heroin. Nicotine, whether supplied in patches or gum, only partially suppresses the withdrawal symptoms caused by smoking cessation[232] (see also Chapter 6). The poor long-term abstinence rate afforded by nicotine replacement leaves no doubt that craving for cigarettes remains, for most smokers, largely unabated. This is especially intriguing in view of the fact that methadone is a heroin surrogate, whereas nicotine is – well – nicotine. If smoking is equated with nicotine consumption, the only possible conclusion is that whereas methadone is an efficient substitute for heroin, nicotine (from "replacement" devices) is a poor substitute for nicotine (from cigarettes). By comparison, acupuncture is a far better nicotine substitute; in fact, it is twice as good as nicotine[677, J]!

If something about the logic of the last sentences seems a bit skewed, the reader may well wonder why it did not seem to have bothered the majority of researchers in this area. It is possible that most researchers are satisfied with the popular explanation (see Chapter 8) that cigarettes are preferred because of their speed of delivery. However, the "nicotine delivery kinetics" theory cannot account for the discrepancies noted here between methadone and nicotine "replacement" treatment. In fact, one of the reasons methadone was chosen as a heroin surrogate was precisely the fact that its onset of action is slow[358].

The discrepancies between "nicotine replacement" treatment, on the one hand, and methadone maintenance treatment, on the other, can easily be reconciled. The observations summarized above appear discrepant only on the assumptions that (1) smoking is a drug addiction, (2) nicotine is the drug in tobacco that causes this addiction, and (3) nicotine addiction is comparable to heroin addiction. All these ostensible discrepancies vanish once smoking is understood to be a habit in which nicotine has no major role, and nicotine is understood to be as similar to heroin as penguins are to fish.

[J]This is particularly interesting considering that a recent meta-analysis of acupuncture techniques for smoking cessation concludes that *"Acupuncture was not superior to sham acupuncture for smoking cessation* (p.393)[704]." This seems to suggest that sham acupuncture is also more effective for smoking cessation than NRT!

4. WHY DOES NRT SUPPRESS WITHDRAWAL SYMPTOMS ALTOGETHER?

The data reviewed so far indicate that "nicotine replacement therapy," despite the powerful suggestion embedded in this term, is a misnomer (hence the double quotes we have been careful to enclose this term with). Unlike methadone maintenance, NRT does not appear to operate by nicotine replacement. Yet, if nicotine deprivation is not the primary reason for the subjective smoking withdrawal reactions in humans, how does NRT suppress these symptoms, albeit only partially? We offer three possible answers, which are not mutually exclusive.

4.1 The Sickness Hypothesis

There are solid reasons to suspect that the suppressant effects of nicotine on smoking withdrawal symptoms may be caused by raising blood nicotine to near toxic levels. This hypothesis is supported by reports that nicotine doses that are 50 percent higher than the habitual doses produce nausea in smokers[131]. Nicotine patches, specifically, can cause nausea and vomiting in up to 40 percent of smokers[e.g.,327]. This hypothesis is discussed in more detail in Chapter 12.

4.2 The Placebo Hypothesis.

In a recent study[238], smokers in acute abstinence received either a cigarette of their regular brand or a de-nicotinized cigarette. The two types of cigarette had the same effect on the onset time, course and intensity of tobacco withdrawal symptoms. Thus, despite the absence of nicotine in the de-nicotinized cigarettes, their effect on withdrawal symptoms was equal to the effect of regular cigarettes. In the same vein, sensory stimulation by a citric acid inhaler in the absence of nicotine reduced subjective withdrawal symptoms[40]. Finally, abstinent smokers who were told that they would receive nicotine gum, but actually received placebo, had significantly less withdrawal symptoms than participants who were told that they would receive placebo[296]. These observations indicate that placebo effects are important determinants of withdrawal suppression by nicotine. Unfortunately, the placebo gums or patches used in most studies do not mimic the effects of nicotine on heart rate[580] and appetite[e.g.,239,326,641]. Consequently, participants can discriminate between the nicotine device and its intended placebo[e.g.,296,479,480], rendering the placebo control in these studies virtually useless.

4.3 The Secondary Reinforcer Hypothesis

As just stated, nicotine produces changes in heart rate and other physiological changes that are familiar to smokers. As these internal cues are normally paired with the pleasurable effects of smoking, they may become secondary reinforcers through classical conditioning. Therefore, when the same cues are elicited by nicotine patches or gum, they may reduce the subjective withdrawal symptoms even if these symptoms are not caused by nicotine deprivation.

5. CONCLUSION

In this short chapter we wanted to make three important points with regard to the so-called nicotine replacement therapies. Firstly, the efficacy of such treatments is very modest, compared to many non-chemical methods of smoking cessation. Secondly, a comparison with methadone maintenance treatment for heroin addiction shows that at no level can the presumed similarity between the two types of treatment be sustained. Hence, our conclusion is that the two types of interventions operate by entirely different mechanisms. Finally, we propose three mechanisms that can account for the modest effect of NRTs on smoking withdrawal. None of these mechanisms requires the assumption that smoking is driven by nicotine addiction. In the next chapter, we revisit the first of these mechanisms, namely the satiation effected by nicotine toxicity.

Chapter 12

THE TALE OF NICOTINE COMPENSATION

1. THE NICOTINE COMPENSATION HYPOTHESIS

When heroin-addicted individuals have access to unlimited supplies of heroin, they will rapidly increase self-administration to many times their usual dose[312]. As mentioned in Chapter 9, cigarette smokers do not display such a continuous upping of intake. The average number of cigarettes consumed daily by smokers is less than 20 in Great Britain[452] and only slightly more than 20 in the USA[665]. Smokers rapidly arrive at their preferred number of cigarettes per day and the number remains stable for years[665,682] and even declines in older smokers[665]. This observation is problematic for the nicotine addiction hypothesis. If nicotine is addictive in the same sense that heroin is, as so frequently claimed by various authorities, smokers should strive to consume as much nicotine as they possibly can.

Even without smoking more cigarettes, smokers could still increase nicotine consumption by switching to cigarettes with a higher nicotine yield. This does not seem to be the case, however. Research on long-term smoking patterns in the population shows exactly the opposite trend. In 1954, the average nicotine/tar level (in milligrams per cigarette) was 2.7/38[283]. Filter cigarettes were introduced in 1954[518] and "low tar" cigarettes were introduced before 1967, when the average nicotine/tar content per cigarette was already half the amount of what it was in 1954 $(1.4/22)^{518}$. In the five years preceding the Surgeon General's Report[665], the average nicotine/tar level per cigarette dropped to one third of the original yield (0.9/13) and remained fairly stable until 1992[283]. Therefore, between 1954 and 1985 the average smoker lost over 60 percent of the nicotine and tar yield of his or her cigarettes.

The observation that smokers do not tend to increase nicotine intake beyond a certain level, either by smoking more cigarettes or by increasing the nicotine yield of their cigarettes can be explained by the toxicity of tobacco smoke constituents, and specifically of nicotine. We shall discuss this point later in the chapter. However, toxicity cannot explain why presumably nicotine-addicted smokers would be willing to accept a *reduction* in nicotine intake when switching to lower-yield brands. This is clearly a problem for the nicotine addiction hypothesis. It could easily be resolved, if smokers compensated for the reduction in nicotine yield by smoking more cigarettes. There is no indication, however, that the average number of cigarettes per smoker increased threefold in the USA between 1951 and 1988, and strong evidence against this notion[449,518,665]. The nicotine compensation hypothesis, which is the focus of the present chapter, attempts to resolve this thorny problem in a different manner. It postulates that as nicotine is the addictive agent that maintains smoking, smokers are unwilling (or unable) to accept reductions in nicotine intake. Consequently, according to the nicotine compensation hypothesis, they will use various strategies to counter any reduction in nicotine intake, primarily by "oversmoking" their cigarettes.

2.   SHORT- AND LONG-TERM SWITCHING STUDIES

Since the beginning of the 1970s, following the introduction of "lighter" cigarettes that were publicized by cigarette manufacturers as less dangerous, extensive research has investigated whether smokers compensate for a reduction in the tar/nicotine yield of their cigarettes by strategies other than increasing the number of cigarettes smoked. Most studies have been short-term laboratory studies in which smokers of high-nicotine, high-tar cigarettes switched to lower yield cigarettes. The more sophisticated studies monitored blood or urine levels of nicotine or cotinine (a stable metabolite of nicotine) in these participants, and measured compensation as deviations from the levels predicted by cigarette yield.

In a study by Zacny and Stitzer[733], for example, ten smokers of a high-yield brand were asked to smoke a different brand of cigarettes each week for 5 weeks. The different brands varied in nicotine yield from 0.1 to 1.1 mg and the order of brands was counterbalanced. On the first and last day of each week, participants smoked two cigarettes of their assigned brand in a laboratory session in which subjective, behavioral and biological measures were taken. This study found that cotinine levels were substantially lower after a week of smoking ultra-light cigarettes when compared to a week of the usual high-yield brand. However, the differences in cotinine levels among the brands were smaller than predicted by the cigarettes' nicotine/tar yield. This finding was accounted for by the observation that the participants smoked more cigarettes and took larger and more closely spaced puffs when smoking the low-yield cigarettes. Notably, as is regularly reported but rarely stressed in such studies, the participants did not like the lower-yield cigarettes: They rated them as being less strong, less hot, less harsh, having less and poorer taste, delivering more air than smoke and being less satisfying. As we shall argue later, this highly typical finding may be crucial for understanding compensatory smoking.

Short-term studies do not control for the possibility that adjusting to a new brand of cigarettes may take time[e.g.,434,507,644], and hence that compensation could just be a temporary phenomenon. Recent long-term studies, however, indicate that whereas smokers seem to adjust gradually – in terms of subjective satisfaction – to the lighter cigarettes[e.g.,190,644,645,699], they still have higher cotinine and nicotine levels than expected from the reduction in nicotine yield of their new brand. This finding has also been reported in other recent studies[e.g.,192,630,709]. Thus, smokers apparently continue to compensate partially for the loss of nicotine/tar yield when switching to lighter brands.

In summary, disregarding variability in methodology and results, most short- and long-term switching studies are fairly consistent. Smokers who switch to lighter cigarettes up-regulate their smoking, mostly by taking larger and more frequent puffs. Other possible strategies, such as "vent" blocking (blocking ventilation holes in filters), leaving shorter cigarette butts, or increasing inhalation, appear to be less common means of compensation[577].

This upregulation of smoking accounts for the finfing that smokers switching to lower-yield brands are found to have higher blood levels of cotinine and nicotine than expected from the reduction in nicotine yield[e.g.,20,92,181,191,555,556,645,662,733].

As mentioned earlier, this finding has been viewed as compelling evidence for the nicotine addiction hypothesis. It would constitute such evidence, however, only if up-regulation of smoking were in fact motivated by the loss of nicotine. This caveat is completely ignored by most researchers, who seem to consider it obvious that smoking up-regulation is determined by nicotine. For example, Woodward and Tunstall-Pedoe[726] concluded *"that smokers appear to self-titrate their consumption of nicotine by more aggressive smoking of lower-strength cigarettes* (p. 821)." Djordjevic *et al.*[144] stated that their results were obtained *"because of smokers' compensation for low nicotine delivery* (p. 2015)." Similarly unqualified inferences are made by many other compensation researchers[e.g.,7,48,66,279,348,349]. As we shall demonstrate, these inferences represent a prevailing bias rather than an empirically based conclusion.

2.1   Compensation for What?

There are two possible scenarios that would be consistent with the thesis that smokers who switch to lighter cigarettes compensate for loss of nicotine. One possibility is that the relatively low doses of nicotine yielded by "light" cigarettes provide less reward compared to the smoker's customary higher-yield brands. In this scenario, smoking up-regulation compensates for loss of positive reinforcement. Alternatively, the mechanism for smoking up-regulation may be similar to that of heroin: if nicotine causes physical dependence, then the reduction of nicotine in the brain produces dysphoric abstinence symptoms, which can be alleviated by further supply of nicotine. In this scenario, nicotine serves as a negative reinforcer and up-regulation is the smokers' way to prevent or counter an aversive nicotine withdrawal syndrome.

In Chapter 8 we reviewed the evidence for the alleged positive reinforcing properties of nicotine in humans. Our review of self-administration studies and experiments using nicotine in the form of injections, gum and transdermal patches concluded that nicotine is not rewarding for non-smokers, and may be a weak reinforcer at best (due to conditioning and placebo effects) for deprived smokers. In this context, we argued that the self-administration studies that were considered "conclusive" by the Surgeon General [264,266] actually reveal that nicotine is no more reinforcing than saline. We also cited nicotine nasal spray experiments[483] in which nicotine-deprived smokers were indifferent to nicotine nasal spray whereas non-deprived smokers significantly preferred nicotine-free spray.

The idea that nicotine, like heroin, produces physical dependence and hence can function as a negative reinforcer was refuted in Chapter 9. Dysphoric withdrawal symptoms in abstaining smokers were blocked by cigarettes without nicotine[e.g.,73,699] but were only partially suppressed by nicotine gum or transdermal patches. More dramatically, not a single ex-smoker, re-exposed to nicotine by wearing nicotine transdermal patches for 12 consecutive weeks, expressed a craving for cigarettes or for transdermal patches following this treatment[508]. Finally, mecamylamine did not produce precipitated abstinence symptoms in heavy smokers[e.g.,162,493].

In summary, nicotine does not seem to have significant positive or negative reinforcing properties in humans, including non-deprived smokers. In the absence of such reinforcing properties, there is every reason to doubt that up-regulation of smoking after switching from high- to low-yield cigarettes is induced by loss of nicotine.

2.2   Up-Regulation for Loss of Taste

The conviction that up-regulation of smoking is motivated by reduced nicotine yield has led to the otherwise incomprehensible fact that the vast majority of studies that used cigarette brand as an independent variable did not attempt to separate the effects of nicotine and tar. This is a very serious methodological omission, as the correlation between tar and nicotine levels in commercial cigarettes is 0.90[550,552]. Therefore, attributing the results of these studies to nicotine, rather than to tar, requires a breathtaking leap of faith. This feat is especially daring in view of the fact that smoking pleasure is determined to a large extent by the sensations in the respiratory tract that accompany smoke inhalation and are caused primarily by tar[541]. In fact, the role of these sensations, and hence of tar, in maintaining smoking is much better established than that of nicotine (see Chapter 8).

Several lines of evidence have established the importance of tar, rather than of nicotine, in determining a variety of smoking parameters. A study by Sutton et al.[645] found that the tar yield of the cigarettes predicted puffing patterns (and hence blood levels of nicotine) to a much higher degree than nicotine. This observation was confirmed by several other investigators[26,57,255,411,529,543,630,680]. Others demonstrated that subjective ratings of satisfaction, pleasantness, harshness or desirability of cigarettes were either unrelated to nicotine content[57,533] or depended on "taste" rather than on the central effects of nicotine[310,450]. Cigarettes equal in tar but higher in nicotine were rated as more satisfying, more enjoyable and stronger in various experiments[25,26,255], but these experiments did not control for nicotine's peripheral sensory action[541]. In a study cited earlier[733], smokers disliked the low-nicotine (and low-tar) cigarettes not because they were lacking in psychoactive effects, but rather because they were lacking in taste. We submit that an objective evaluation of these data, together with the wealth of evidence cited in Chapter 8 for the importance of sensory stimulation in smoking, lead to the conclusion that short-term smoking up-regulation is not motivated by the need to compensate for loss of nicotine in the brain. Rather, the main motivation is to compensate for the reduction in "taste" and in other pleasurable aspects of smoking, which are produced primarily by tar and to a lesser extent by the peripheral action of nicotine. Further support for this claim comes from cross-sectional studies of smoking parameters.

3.   CROSS-SECTIONAL "COMPENSATION" STUDIES

A third empirical approach to nicotine compensation, in addition to short- and long-term switching studies, has been cross-sectional designs. In these studies, the nicotine/tar levels are not manipulated by switching from high-yield to low-yield cigarettes. Instead, cotinine and nicotine blood levels in habitual smokers of high nicotine/tar cigarettes are compared to the same parameters in smokers of low-yield brands[e.g.,44,47,65,154,228,282,348,405,532,553,726].

Most studies report that the nicotine intake of smokers of "lighter" brands (as evident from blood levels of cotinine and nicotine) is lower than that of smokers of high nicotine/tar yield. However, as in short- and long-term switching studies, all studies but one[532] found that the discrepancy between the two groups in blood nicotine and cotinine levels could not be fully accounted for by the difference in the cigarettes' nicotine yield. Specifically, smokers of "light" cigarettes had higher blood levels of nicotine or cotinine than would be expected by the nicotine yield of these brands. In the vast majority of cross-sectional studies, this discrepancy between predicted and observed differences in blood nicotine and cotinine levels was taken as evidence for compensation[e.g.,7,48,65,66,144,154,228,278,282,348,405,486,552,553,726]. This inference, however, is entirely without basis.

The term "compensation" implies a process by which smokers up-regulate smoking as a maneuver aimed to counteract a reduction in nicotine levels. The compensation hypothesis holds that when smokers, who are purportedly addicted to nicotine, switch to lower yield cigarettes, they attempt to maintain the level of nicotine they had been accustomed to by over-smoking their cigarettes. Therefore, as noted also in a recent review of the compensation literature[577], this term can be meaningfully used only in reference to smokers who switch from high nicotine/tar cigarettes to lower nicotine/tar cigarettes. Whereas short- and long-term switching studies are valid methods for examining compensation, findings of cross-sectional studies reflect compensation only if the smokers of lower-yield brand in these studies have switched from higher-yield brand. Among the studies we reviewed, however, *not one* provided evidence that the participants had indeed switched from high-yield to lower yield brands. In fact, it is very unlikely that the differences found in cross-sectional studies between smokers of high- and low-yield cigarettes can be attributed to compensation in the sense implied above.

As mentioned earlier, between 1955 and 1983 the average nicotine/tar yield of cigarettes was reduced three-fold. Given that most smokers start smoking at or after the age of fifteen, the vast majority of smokers born before 1968 have experienced a reduction in the yield of their cigarettes over time. This trend continued after 1983. In 1986, for example, 9.2 percent of all adult smokers switched brands[607] and about 26 percent of switching smokers turned to a lighter brand[495]. Thus, even amongst smokers younger than 30 years of age, many have probably switched to lighter brands and would therefore be expected to compensate.

But not all smokers are switchers. A large number of the younger participants in the cross-sectional studies (most published between 1982 and

1995) can be assumed to have started their smoking habit on low nicotine/tar cigarettes and therefore could not be compensating for cigarettes with higher levels of these compounds. Participants in one study[282], for example, had a mean age of 27–29 years and had smoked, on an average, for 10–12 years. These participants had reached smoking age when "light" or "medium" cigarettes were common (after 1978). Yet, the authors of this and other cross-sectional studies explain differences between smokers of "light" and "heavy" cigarettes as partial compensation by the first group, without presenting any evidence that smokers in this group had ever smoked higher-yield cigarettes in the past.

If the differences obtained in cross-sectional studies are due to compensation for loss of nicotine, then switchers from high-yield to lower yield cigarettes should have higher blood cotinine and nicotine levels than smokers who have always smoked low-yield cigarettes. Though this seems an obvious deduction that could be easily tested, we found only one study that addressed it directly[348]. This study found that switchers had higher urine cotinine levels than smokers who had always smoked low-yield cigarettes. However, the switchers in this study smoked roughly 60 percent more cigarettes than participants who had always smoked light cigarettes (14.9 versus 9.1 cigarettes per day), completely accounting for the difference in observed urine cotinine levels. In this study, therefore, switchers and smokers who never switched extracted similar amounts of nicotine from their cigarettes, a finding that contradicts the compensation hypothesis.

Indirect evidence for nicotine compensation in cross-sectional studies could be gleaned by comparing blood levels of nicotine or cotinine between cohorts of different ages. If the youngest cohort, which is most likely to have never switched, would have lower levels of blood nicotine and cotinine, yet smoked the same amount of the same brand of cigarettes as older smokers, this would be consistent with a process of compensation. Only four cross-sectional studies provided age-related information. Two of those did not find an age effect[282,532]. Bridges et al.[65] found that younger smokers had lower blood nicotine and cotinine levels than older ones, but the older smokers consumed more high-yield (non-filter) cigarettes than the younger smokers. Hill et al.[278] found that smokers aged 18–24 years had lower plasma cotinine levels than older smokers, but did not report whether these smokers smoked the same amount and/or the same yield cigarettes as the older smokers. Thus, this line of research did not produce any evidence for the compensation hypothesis.

3.1   Down-Regulation of Smoking: Compensation Turned on its Head

As stated earlier, the differences found in cross-sectional studies between nicotine and cotinine levels of high- versus low-yield smokers have been universally attributed the process of compensation, which follows switching from higher- to lower-yield cigarettes. This inference, which unwittingly begs the question of nicotine addiction, is unwarranted by available evidence; in fact, as we shall presently illustrate, it is plainly inconsistent with well-known facts. Nevertheless, it represents an almost universal prejudice that has biased the interpretation of most cross-sectional studies.

Specifically, in all cross-sectional studies, cotinine blood levels in smokers of low nicotine/tar cigarettes are predicted by using smokers of high nicotine/tar cigarettes as a reference point. Thus, if a given brand of high-yield cigarettes contains 1.0 mg nicotine and a given low-yield cigarette contains 0.5 mg nicotine, cotinine levels of the smokers of the low-yield brand are expected to be 50 percent lower than those of the high-yield smokers. If they are only 25 percent lower, the smokers of the lower-yield brand are said to "compensate" or "up-regulate" by 50 percent. However, if the researchers had used the smokers of low-yield cigarettes as a reference point, they would have concluded that the smokers of high-yield cigarettes are *down-regulating* their nicotine intake. We submit that there is no *a priori* reason, besides the seductive bias introduced by the compensation hypothesis, to prefer the former interpretation.

Down-regulation of smoking when switching from low- to high-yield cigarettes has been consistently found in switching studies[e.g.,48,123,273,279,509,658]. This effect has been relatively de-emphasized, as switching studies were primarily designed to examine whether reduced tar/nicotine cigarettes were an effective means of curtailing the intake of tobacco smoke. Therefore, the authors of these studies were primarily interested in demonstrating compensation for lower yield. However, a recent review[577] found that down-regulation of smoking is in fact a much larger effect than up-regulation. The mean effect size for up-regulation when switching to a lower-yield brand in switching studies was in the order of 50 percent, whereas the effect size for down-regulation when switching to a higher-yield brand was 80 percent, a statistically significant difference. This finding opens the door to an entirely different interpretation of this body of data, specifically regarding the role of nicotine in regulating smoking.

4.   NICOTINE'S ROLE IN LIMITING SMOKING: PHARMACODYNAMIC SATIATION

High doses of nicotine in humans produce toxicity, manifested by nausea, vomiting, diarrhea, abdominal pain[e.g.,431,565,728], seizures[e.g.,610,727] and even death[e.g.,647]. Indeed, nicotine is sometimes used in suicide attempts[431,565,727].

Even low doses of nicotine can produce adverse effects. When nicotine is administered subcutaneously[184], by gum[434] or by transdermal patches[e.g.,327,617,626], it produces nausea and vomiting not only in non-smokers[184,626] but also in up to 41 percent of smokers[327,617]. Though considerable tolerance to these effects develops over time, it is not complete. As mentioned earlier, increasing smoking by 50 percent induced nausea in smokers[131] and nicotine in nasal spray was aversive to smokers when it followed their usual daily number of cigarettes [483].

There is substantial support for the idea that the effect of nicotine is to *limit*, rather than to facilitate, smoking. As discussed above, when smokers switch to cigarettes with higher nicotine and tar yield they down-regulate their smoking. In addition, several studies examined the effect of applying nicotine before or during smoking by intravenous injections[e.g.,45,551], gum[e.g.,155,274], patches[e.g.,185,539], oral capsules[e.g.,110,698] or nasal spray[482]. The majority of these studies showed partial down-regulation of smoking (see Scherer[577], for review). In a recent study by Benowitz et al.[49], transdermal nicotine patches releasing up to three times the doses recommended to facilitate cessation were applied to heavy smokers who were not interested in quitting smoking. The number of cigarettes smoked and the nicotine absorbed from these cigarettes declined by approximately 30 and 40 percent, respectively. The authors concluded: *"The dose-suppression curve is hyperbolic, suggesting that there is a dose of nicotine, not far exceeding the highest dose in our study, that would have almost completely suppressed nicotine intake* (p. 961)." This study, together with the earlier ones, not only confirms that nicotine is an agent that limits smoking. It also suggests that there exists an individual, or possibly an absolute, ceiling of blood nicotine levels beyond which further intake of nicotine becomes so aversive as to deter even the most avid smoker.

Gori and Lynch[228] provided additional evidence for this contention. They discovered that a ceiling in plasma nicotine and cotinine levels was reached when about 20 cigarettes were smoked per day. This ceiling was not exceeded significantly even when smokers consumed up to 60 cigarettes per day. The authors suggested (p. 321) *"that the limiting factor is probably nicotine intake itself, since plasma nicotine and cotinine values display similar ceilings, while the nicotine to cotinine conversion rate remains constant."* They termed this phenomenon **"pharmacodynamic satiation."** Similarly, Hill and his coworkers[278] showed that nicotine and cotinine blood levels reached a plateau when more than 21 cigarettes per day were consumed. These findings, together with those of Benowitz et al.[49], imply that there may be an absolute ceiling for nicotine satiation in spite of the partial tolerance that develops to its toxicity.

The average smoker reaches reaches pharmacodynamic satiation with about 20 cigarettes per day. This figure coincides approximately with the number of cigarettes consumed by the average smoker both in England[452] and the USA[665]. Although this average means that many smokers light more than 20 cigarettes daily, even those who smoke 30[278] or even 60[228] cigarettes per day do not extract much more nicotine from their cigarettes than those who smoke 20. Therefore, heavy smokers must be down-regulating their smoking to a considerable extent. This down-regulation is apparently motivated by the toxicity of nicotine and, perhaps, of other smoke constituents. As we elaborate below, the hypothesis that nicotine limits smoking provides an alternative account for the (modest) utility of "nicotine replacement" devices for smoking cessation

4.1   A Satiation Account of "Nicotine Replacement Therapy"

As noted in the previous chapter, the rationale for so-called nicotine replacement treatments was the same as for methadone maintenance treatment for opiate addiction. A comparison between the two treatments, however, indicates that their mechanisms of action are different. This comparison, together with the meager efficacy of "nicotine replacement" treatments, undermines the nicotine addiction hypothesis on which these treatments were based.

At this point, we can elaborate on one of the alternative explanations suggested in Chapter 11 for the effects of nicotine gum and patches on smoking cessation. This explanation, like the other two suggested in Chapter 11, has nothing to do with "replacement" and does not depend on the validity of the nicotine addiction hypothesis. Specifically, we suggest that pre-loading smokers with nicotine simply brings them closer to the toxicity ceiling, where any more nicotine will be aversive. Hence, smokers will down-regulate by smoking fewer cigarettes and by under-smoking their cigarettes, thus weakening the behavioral habit and facilitating quitting. As aversion for nicotine is incompatible with craving for cigarettes, both craving and relapse will be reduced by nicotine releasing devices such as nicotine transdermal patches and nicotine gum.

This "satiation" account of the effectiveness of nicotine gum and patches is much more consistent with the evidence cited in this book than the "replacement" account, which is based on the presumed similarity between nicotine and heroin. In particular, it accounts for the limited efficacy of NRTs, as documented in the previous chapter. Under the nicotine addiction account, it is rather mystifying to discover that smokers do not quit smoking despite receiving their presumed drug of choice through gums or patches. The puzzle resolves itself if the satiation account is substituted for the "replacement" account: Superimposed nicotine reduces smoking by making it aversive, but as smokers do not smoke to acquire nicotine, it cannot provide an acceptable alternative to smoking.

5. SUMMARY: THE ROLE OF NICOTINE IN SMOKING TITRATION

The fact that smokers tend to maintain a stable level of smoking, both by smoking a relatively invariant number of cigarettes and by partially up- and down-regulating their smoking in response to the tar/nicotine yield of their cigarettes, has been recognized for many years. Not unexpectedly, both up- and down-regulation have been almost universally attributed to nicotine[e.g.,48,279,348,349,416,726], so much so that smoking titration has been commonly referred to as "nicotine titration." For example, Kolonen et al.[349] wrote that *"smokers seem to up- or down-regulate their smoke intake by changing puff volume and inhalation to maintain their usual levels of blood nicotine (p. 704)."* The same unquestioned assumption is evident in the conclusions of Hill and Marquardt[279]: *"Assay of urinary and plasma cotinine levels in smokers smoking brands with different nicotine content showed that smokers adjust their smoking habits to maintain a constant level of nicotine. This self-titration of nicotine may pose a health hazard even with relatively low-nicotine cigarettes (p. 652)."* These assumptions must have been so self-evident to the authors (and perhaps the journal editors) that they did not find it necessary to qualify them anywhere. This is another example of the prevailing "nicotine bias" we have referred to repeatedly throughout this book. An objective scientist would refrain from stating unequivocally that the observed titration is a strategy aimed to maintain nicotine level. It is a different matter to report an observation than to suggest an interpretation, but in this field of research, this distinction is rarely observed.

The evidence we have reviewed so far suggests that "nicotine titration" is a misnomer. Specifically, up- and down-regulation of smoking are not symmetrical processes. While nicotine seems to be involved in down-regulation, as most researchers agree, it does not seem to have a role in up-regulation. Instead, up-regulation appears to be motivated by other aspects of the smoking habit, primarily by the sensory rewards of smoking. The evidence reviewed here indicates that "light" cigarettes are smoked more intensely because of their reduced tar, "taste," and other sensory qualities, not because of a reduction in psychoactive effects supposedly incurred by the low nicotine yield.

In summary, neither "nicotine compensation" nor "nicotine titration" are sustained by empirical evidence; hence, neither has any bearing on the nicotine addiction hypothesis. Both terms reflect a pervasive bias in the smoking literature, which attributes an unwarranted role to nicotine in determining smoking. Paradoxically, a review of the evidence suggests that the main role nicotine has in determining smoking may be in imposing a ceiling on the extent or intensity of smoking. This effect is due not to the purported addictive properties of nicotine, but rather to its toxic effects.

Chapter 13

EPILOGUE

1.   IS NICOTINE AN ADDICTIVE DRUG? CONCLUSION

This book reviewed and evaluated the evidence for the Surgeon General's influential declaration[665] (p. 9) that *"Cigarettes and other forms of tobacco are addicting,"* that *"Nicotine is the drug in tobacco that causes addiction,"* and that *"The pharmacologic and behavioral processes that determine tobacco addiction are similar to those that determine addiction to drugs such as heroin and cocaine."* Although this assertion has been almost universally adopted by the scientific community, government agencies, the media and the public, we found that it is not sustained by empirical evidence. Instead, our analysis of the research to date indicates that if nicotine contributes to the persistence of smoking, it is not due to its purportedly gratifying psychoactive properties but rather to its contribution to the "taste" of inhaled smoke and perhaps to placebo effects and acquired (secondary) reinforcing properties in experienced smokers. Thus, nicotine's role in maintaining the smoking habit bears no similarity to the role played by genuinely addictive drugs such as heroin, barbiturates, alcohol or other drugs to which nicotine is routinely compared.

In contrast to the case of heroin or cocaine, there exists no convincing demonstration that animals will *initiate* self-administration of nicotine. Moreover, even a demonstration that animals will *maintain* nicotine self-administration can only be achieved by extremely dubious manipulations of the procedure. The conditions that were imposed to induce animals to maintain self-administration of nicotine included food restriction or deprivation, prior conditioning to food or drugs, simultaneous administration of additional reinforcers, restraining, and prior nicotine administration. Remarkably, even under these facilitatory manipulations, a large proportion of the animals were excluded from analysis in many studies for failing to self-administer nicotine. In addition, most studies did not employ adequate controls to rule out plausible, or even obvious, alternative explanations for the results observed under these conditions. Only a handful of studies included "yoked" controls, and even an elementary saline control group to control for nicotine's effect on activation and learning was lacking in the vast majority of studies. Consequently, effects that were attributed to nicotine's reinforcing effects in these studies are much more likely to have reflected other factors, primarily a lack of extinction of prior learning driven by food or drugs like cocaine and the activating effects of nicotine. This conclusion is supported by the few studies that did employ appropriate controls. In addition, conditioned place preference and conditioned taste preference studies fail to demonstrate that animals "like" the effects of nicotine. Thus, the idea that nicotine is reinforcing to animals is not convincingly supported by experimental evidence.

A similar picture arose when we scrutinized the evidence for the contention that nicotine has reinforcing effects in humans, effects that are widely believed to maintain the habit of smoking (see Chapter 8). While nicotine surely has psychoactive effects, those effects seem to be primarily unpleasant. Without exception and independently of route of administration, nicotine was found to be aversive to non-smokers. Only a minority of studies found nicotine reinforcing to deprived smokers. Few if any of these studies recognized that inert placebo manipulations are inadequate for smokers, whose ability to identify the "taste" of nicotine and its physiological effects is well-established. Consequently, they lacked appropriate control groups to rule out the possibility that these reinforcing effects were due to placebo effects. Even so, most studies showed that pure nicotine has no reinforcing properties for smokers or that they distinctly dislike its effects. Thus, it is inconceivable that the psychoactive effects of nicotine constitute a reason for smoking. Paradoxically, our analysis of the "nicotine compensation" research indicates that nicotine has a much more prominent role in *limiting*, rather than in perpetuating, tobacco smoking.

In sharp contrast to the case of heroin or other addictive drugs, neither animals nor humans show long-term increases in nicotine consumption in any form. If any age-related long-term changes are discernible in smoking prevalence, they all point in the opposite direction. Therefore, if nicotine has any reinforcing effects, as the nicotine addiction thesis maintains, no tolerance to these effects develops over time. Initial increases in the consumption of cigarettes in the novice smoker coincide with and are indistinguishable from the concomitant development of tolerance to the (well-established) aversive effects of nicotine.

A nicotine abstinence syndrome, which is believed to indicate the development of physical dependence, has been reported both in animals and humans. However, the abstinence syndrome in rats is not dysphoric (it may be even pleasurable according to the conditioned taste aversion paradigm), hence it cannot motivate further consumption of nicotine. Furthermore, there is no indication that the abstinence syndrome observed in rats is relevant to humans. As discussed in Chapter 9, the abstinence syndrome in humans has been dissociated experimentally into a nicotine-specific withdrawal syndrome, which is not dysphoric, and other reactions that are known to follow the interruption of many habits in which no psychoactive drugs are involved. Moreover, unlike opiate antagonists in heroin addicts, the nicotine antagonists mecamylamine does not precipitate a withdrawal syndrome in smokers, a finding that negates the existence of physical dependence on nicotine. Finally, there are no known instances that prolonged use of pure nicotine causes physical dependence. To the contrary, twelve weeks of sustained nicotine absorption via transdermal patches failed to induce nicotine craving in never-smokers and ex-smokers alike.

In summary, even according to the lenient modern criteria of drug addiction[665,711], which do not require physical dependence, nicotine is not an addictive drug. The evidence available to us contradicts the accepted notion that nicotine is a major determinant of the persistence of smoking, or that its presence in tobacco smoke increases the difficulty of quitting the habit. Ironically, there is substantial evidence that nicotine may in fact limit smoking due to its toxic effects.

1.1   On the Purported Similarity between Nicotine and Heroin

The Surgeon General's statement to the effect the nicotine and heroin are similarly addictive has been canonized by others[e.g.,269,657] and popularized into a smoke-talk cliché. The evidence reviewed in this book shows this equation to be nothing less than preposterous. Table 13.1 summarizes the major differences between the relevant attributes of nicotine and heroin.

Table 13.1 A comparison between the attributes of nicotine and heroin

Attributes	Nicotine	Heroin
Unconditional self-administration in pure form by animals	No	Yes
Conditioned place preference in animals	No	Yes
Unconditional self-administration in pure form by humans	No	Yes
Administration induces pleasant sensations or positive mood	No	Yes
Tolerance to reinforcing effect)	No	Yes
Dysphoric drug-specific abstinence syndrome in animals	No	Yes
Increased lever-pressing for lower effective doses of drug	No	Yes
Dysphoric drug specific abstinence syndrome in humans	No	Yes
Precipitated abstinence syndrome in humans	No	Yes
Replacement therapy abolishes abstinence syndrome	No	Yes
Re-addiction after long-term exposure to pure drug in humans	No	Yes*
Craving for drug after long-term exposure or re-exposure to pure drug	No	Yes
Replacement therapy prevents consumption of the target drug	No	Yes
Consumption persists in spite of current legal restrictions	No	Yes
Population prevalence remains unchanged compared to 40 years ago	No	Yes
* Not tested directly, but assumed		

Most of the differences between heroin and nicotine that are summarized in Table 13.1 pertain to operational definitions of current criteria for drug dependence[87,665,711]. The rest of the items are descriptions of *"The pharmacologic and behavioral processes that determine tobacco addiction,"* which are supposed to be *"similar to those that determine addiction to drugs such as heroin and cocaine* (p. 9)[665]." As this table demonstrates, the alleged similarity of nicotine to heroin is not supported by any relevant observations. The mere fact that pure nicotine is available over the counter at drugstores in many countries, whereas the purchase of heroine (even in "slow-release" forms!) is a criminal offence, should have caused people to pause and wonder about the equation between nicotine and heroin. That this alleged similarity is nevertheless repeated by scientists, government authorities and the media testifies that nicotine addiction is no longer a conjecture that can be refuted by either evidence or common sense.

2.   WHAT WENT WRONG IN NICOTINE ADDICTION RESEARCH

Our colleagues are no less qualified than ourselves, and many are probably better qualified, to evaluate the research on nicotine addiction. Yet, when we began to scrutinize their reports, we became aware that we not only disagreed with their conclusions, but very often, too often, with their methodology. We are aware of the fact that most scientific reports – including ours, of course – are imperfect. However, the flaws we found in the nicotine research literature are of such magnitude and occur in such a regular fashion that they demand an explanation. A partial list of the methodological shortcomings compiled in this book includes:

- Systematic exclusion of subjects from statistical analyses
- Absence of saline control groups for injected drugs
- Result-biased selection of number of sessions to test manipulations
- Absence of statistical comparisons
- Presenting non-significant results as significant, quasi-synonymously called "reliable"
- A-posteriori selection of statistical comparisons without rationale
- Incomplete reporting of the results of control groups
- Inadequate controls for placebo effects
- Inclusion of selected results from earlier published experiments into new ones without rationale
- Omitting adequate controls for known side-effects of drugs
- Providing two reinforcers but controlling for the effects of only one of them
- Administering "priming" injections to self-administering animals without adequate controls

•   Using previously conditioned animals without controlling for carry-over effects

These methodological flaws have been addressed in detail throughout the book.   In none of the original research reports have we seen any acknowledgement of these shortcomings or their implications for the validity or generality of the results.   Moreover, very few of the reviews that summarized these reports alluded to any of the problems listed above.   A 1988 review of intravenous self-administration studies[217] may exemplify this spirit of uncritical evaluation. The authors state (p. 228): "*If a drug appears to function as a reinforcer, there are several criteria that are commonly applied to assess its effectiveness. These are as follows:*

The absolute rates of responding maintained by the drug in question, expressed as responses by unit time, are of a similar magnitude to those by known drugs of abuse and by non-drug events such as food presentation.

The temporal patterns of responding maintained by the drug are similar to those characteristically maintained under the particular schedule of reinforcement by other drugs of abuse such as cocaine or by non-drug events such as food presentation.

Rates of responding show systematic changes as the dose of the drug is varied.

The rate of responding maintained by the drug is appreciably greater than that maintained by the saline vehicle alone.

Rates of responding maintained by the drug are reduced to near vehicle levels after pretreatment with specific antagonists.

Sufficient amounts of drugs are self-administered to produce gross behavioral or physiological effects.

These criteria provide a uniform basis for comparing results of studies performed in different species and under a variety of conditions."

Thus, the authors of this scholarly review saw no need to even mention the need to exclude confounding effects of nicotine. If nicotine would cause spastic contractions of the muscles controlling the subjects' limb that presses the lever and thus maintain self-administration, then according to these criteria nicotine would be considered a reinforcer. As discussed earlier, the same lack of enthusiasm for critical evaluation is apparent in the Report of the Surgeon General. In reaching its conclusion that "*nicotine satisfied all the criteria discussed in Chapter V as an effective reinforcer* (p.189)," the authors of this report were clearly unruffled by the multitude of methodological flaws listed in this book.

A recent report, entitled *"Nicotine Addiction in Britain*[657]*,"* may be considered an updated British counterpart to the Surgeon General's report, and is characterized by an even more blatant lack of objectivity. We shall give one example, but similar (and much worse) examples are abundant in this scholarly volume. Under the title *"Nicotine self-administration in rats* (p. 47)" the Tobacco Advisory Group of the Royal College of Physicians states the following (references omitted): *"In 1989, Corrigall and Coen succeeded in developing a rat model for nicotine IVSA* [intravenous self-administration]. *The rats learnt to press to obtain IV infusions of nicotine, but did not press an inactive (control) lever in the same test chamber. The rate of lever pressing was related to the dose of nicotine, and the lever pressing ceased if nicotine was no longer available. As in the experiments in monkeys and dogs mentioned above, the lever-pressing produced nicotine and no other substance. The nicotine served as a goal object (positive reinforcer) for these animals, much in the same way as other drugs of abuse and natural rewards. (...) These observations have been reproduced and extended in numerous published experiments from many different laboratories. All these studies demonstrate that rats will self-administer pure nicotine in the absence of any other reward. The validity of the observation is supported by the finding that the plasma concentration of nicotine in rats during IVSA experiments can be close to that in heavy cigarette smokers who inhale."*

The statements, *"The rats learnt to press to obtain IV infusions of nicotine," "All these studies demonstrate that rats will self-administer pure nicotine in the absence of any other reward,"* and *"As in the experiments in monkeys and dogs mentioned above, the lever-pressing produced nicotine and no other substance,"* are, put as mildly as possible, serious distortions of the facts. Please reread Chapter 6 for a detailed discussion of these experiments and, if possible, the actual experiments. The rats in Corrigall and Coen's[115] study, as well as in its replications, did *not* learn to press to obtain IV infusions of nicotine. They learned to do so for *food*. In the only experiment that used a saline control group[31], lever-pressing rates for nicotine and saline in the FR1 schedule did not differ. In other words, in the FR1 schedule animals did not learn to press for nicotine any more than they did for saline. The *"monkeys and dogs mentioned above"* had nearly all learned to press a lever when that lever produced cocaine or other drugs. Thus, *"the lever-pressing produced nicotine and no other substance"* is only true for the period after the animals were switched to nicotine. The British physicians also failed to mention that most of the experiments that *"reproduced and extended"* Corrigall and Coen's 1989 study achieved this feat by excluding up to 40% (and sometimes even more) of the subjects – those that failed to cooperate. Specifically, the study that supposedly found that *"the plasma concentration of nicotine in rats during IVSA experiments can be close to that in heavy cigarette smokers"*[603] excluded 25, 50, and 83 percent (!) of the animals in three respective experimental groups for not showing the desired self-administration behavior. One cannot avoid the impression that both the Surgeon General's report and its British counterpart were aimed as authoritative anti-smoking manifestos rather than objective scientific analyses of the nicotine addiction research.

2.1   The Pitfalls of Near-Consensus

The uncritical endorsement of the nicotine addiction hypothesis by the Surgeon General or the Royal College of Physicians does not explain the low quality of research that scientists in this area have produced. Why did our scholarly colleagues commit such errors? How could they have been so blind to the methodological shortcomings of their own studies? We believe that the primary reason for this state of affairs has to do with the "near-consensus" amongst investigators in this area that nicotine is addictive, a near-consensus that was "enshrined," in the words of Stolerman and Jarvis[635], in the Surgeon General's 1988 report.

One problem created by near-consensus in science is economic in nature. In universities and research centers, publications are the major criterion for tenure and promotion. Therefore, acceptance of articles into mainstream journals and procuring of grant support for one's research has real and immediate economic consequences. In a field dominated by consensus, scientists would naturally prefer to write grant applications and articles that are safely in line with the consensus. It might be easier, for example, to receive grant support for research proposing to corroborate the addictive nature of nicotine than for a proposal aimed to counter this hypothesis or to explore the potentially beneficial properties of nicotine. Research on conformity has demonstrated that consensus stifles not only the *expression* of opposing views, but also non-conforming beliefs and perception, even when objective reality clearly contradicts the "enshrined" view[18]. When opposing the consensus may result in economic sanctions, the power of consensus to coerce intellectual conformity is multiplied.

As the reader is probably aware, scientific papers submitted for publication and grant applications aimed to obtain financial support for research are typically peer-reviewed. Generally, peer review maximizes the probability that experimental flaws would be detected, as even if the authors themselves are well-qualified, their peers presumably share neither the emotional investment nor the theoretical biases that may blind the researchers to methodological flaws or to alternative explanations of their data. Furthermore, the reliance on several reviewers rather than on a single authority is designed to guarantee plurality of opinions and allow for a diversity of theoretical approaches and creative designs. These essential attributes of peer review, however, are threatened or nullified when a research field is under the spell of "near-consensus."

Consensus suppresses skepticism by creating a common theoretical bias towards expected results. If the investigator and his or her referees share a common bias, peer review loses its advantage, as the referees are likely to be as blind towards methodological flaws as the experimenter is. When results are in line with the accepted theory, no alternative accounts of the data are considered, and both researcher and referee are likely to consider the predicted results as validating the experimental procedure. Together, these dynamics of near-consensus all but guarantee the stifling of criticism, suppression of novel ideas and proliferation of sub-standard research. That is one of the reasons that modern philosophy of science considers plurality of views and competition among research programs an essential attribute of the scientific enterprise[e.g.,365].

As Stolerman and Jarvis[635] note, the 1988 Report of the Surgeon General was born out of near-consensus. This fact, by itself, should have cautioned every scientist contributing to this report or reviewing it to be extra-critical in evaluating the experimental data before reaching hasty conclusions. The fact that the report is everything but critical may be attributable to the fact that pivotal sections of the Report were not peer-reviewed at all, at least not in the usual sense of the word.

We have already discussed the brief section entitled: "*Human Studies of Nicotine as a Reinforcer*[665](p. 192)." We showed that amongst six publications cited to support its conclusion, only two were peer-reviewed articles that permit evaluation of their methodology. We have closely scrutinized these two articles (Chapter 8), and found that they exemplify almost every aspect of the deficient scientific standards that characterize the nicotine addiction research. The Surgeon General's report, however, evaluated these studies quite differently, stating that they "*demonstrated conclusively that nicotine itself can serve as an effective reinforcer in humans* (p. 192)." One explanation for the discrepancy between our perception of this work and the Surgeon General's evaluation may be unrelated to the scientific merit of these articles. As the reader may have noticed earlier, one researcher was an author in all six publications, and another co-authored five of them. In the Surgeon General's report, both authors are mentioned under the heading "*The following individuals prepared draft chapters or portions of the Report* (p. ix)" and in addition, one of authors is listed as one of four Scientific Editors of the report. Thus, in this case the same individuals that wrote the original articles may well have been involved in evaluating these articles for the Surgeon General's report and in writing the section that was based on their own studies. In such an intimate setting, genuine peer review is impossible and the conclusion of the Surgeon General cited above is no longer surprising. Moreover, once this conclusion was endorsed by the authority of the Surgeon General, future readers are unlikely to ever return to critique the original reports, and the statement that nicotine is reinforcing in humans is thus "enshrined."

2.2 Science and Morals in Nicotine Addiction Research

One of the meanings of "*enshrine*," according to the Random House College Dictionary[513], is "*to cherish as sacred*." In principle, nothing should be sacred in science except personal integrity, objectivity, skepticism, transparency and, perhaps, the principle that nothing should be sacred in science. This has not always been the case, however, as Kary Mullis, the 1993 laureate of the Nobel Prize in Chemistry, describes in his rather informal style[437]:

"Robert Boyle, who was a Christian and a friend of the English monarch Charles II, made a vacuum pump in the seventeenth century and showed that he could extinguish a candle by pumping the air out of the jar wherein the candle was burning. According to Boyle, whatever was left in the jar after the candle went out constituted a vacuum. In the common vernacular, it meant that absolutely nothing was there. Whether God was in there or not was not something Boyle addressed. He did not know how to measure the existence of God. The religious issue was not as interesting as the issue of what he could measure. The Catholics seriously disagreed. They had documents which clearly stated that God was everywhere. Even some garbage from mistranslations of Aristotle that said "Nature abhorred a vacuum" was taken to mean that Nature just fucking wouldn't allow one at all and that Boyle was an idiot. But the candle went out. Boyle didn't care whether God was there or not because he couldn't measure God. That's when science started to take off. (…)

People who accepted the existence of a vacuum gave their allegiance to the king; people who believed the creation of a vacuum was impossible supported the pope. In 1662, Charles II chartered the Royal Society of London for the Improvement of Natural Knowledge. Boyle was one of the founding members. Those interested in scientific discovery were invited to the Royal Society to demonstrate how things worked. It was thought that through use of this scientific method that science was separated from religion and philosophy, and that included morality. Science freed of morality began to shine".

When Popes, throughout history, were unable to cope with the heretical arguments appearing in published form, they added such publications to the *"Index Librorum Prohibitorum"* – the list of prohibited books. As scientific popes do not officially exist, and there is no formal list of theses that scientists must not question, there is no equivalent "index" in science. However, as described above, there are strong pressures within the scientific community to avoid attacking certain theories, of which the "enshrined" nicotine addiction hypothesis is a prime example. The pressure to conform to this particular theory, in addition to the reasons stated earlier, is that the thesis of nicotine addiction resonates with heavy moral overtones.

The word 'addiction' (see Chapter 2) is highly charged with morality and values, as Akers noted in his brilliant essay, entitled *"Addiction: The Troublesome Concept*[8]*:" "Anything addictive is bad; if it is not addictive, it* *is probably not too bad. A tobacco smoking habit is bad enough, but it is even worse when one thinks of it as an addiction* (p. 778)." According to Goode[224], the negative connotations of the word 'addiction' were the primary reason for widening the scope of this term to include as many harmful habits as possible. In Goode's rather sharp words, "*the scientists and physicians who devised the new terminology of "dependence" were in effect disseminating propaganda to convince the public that nonaddicting substances were just as "bad" for them, that they could be just as dependent on them as on the truly "addicting" drugs* (p. 47)." Even authorities that represent the mainstream of the nicotine addiction position admit that the changes in the definition of addiction were not based on scientific considerations alone. According to the report of the Royal College of Physicians[657], for example, these concepts are "*socially and scientifically defined in that their meaning can be, and has been, changed to reflect changing perceptions rather than to identify unequivocally an invariant, objectively defined entity* (p. 83)."

As discussed above, several factors are liable to discourage scientists from embarking on a research program that stands in opposition to the cherished view. When this view is the official position of government agencies such as the Surgeon General or the National Institute of Drug Abuse, the stakes involved in adopting a skeptic position are especially high. In the case of the nicotine addiction hypothesis, its social and moral connotations increase even further the hesitance of researchers to explore dissenting views. Clearly, opposing the nicotine addiction hypothesis is decidedly *not* politically correct. As mentioned in the introduction, a number of colleagues reacted to our views as if they were tantamount to an endorsement of smoking or a vote of support for the tobacco industry. Thus, the nicotine addiction hypothesis is protected from attempts of refutation by powerful forces, only the minority of which is scientific in nature. The sum total of these forces creates a situation in which scientists are very reluctant to examine this hypothesis critically.

3.   A PLEA FOR DISENSHRINEMENT

"*Scientists*," according to Lakatos[364] "*have thick skins. They do not abandon a theory merely because facts contradict it. They normally either invent some rescue hypothesis to explain what they then call a mere anomaly or, if they cannot explain the anomaly, they ignore it, and direct their attention to other problems* (p. 4)." The area of nicotine addiction research is rich in "rescue hypotheses" and "ignored anomalies." A typical example of a "rescue hypothesis" is the postulation that the lack of complete suppression of smoking withdrawal symptoms by nicotine gum or transdermal patches is due to insufficient nicotine delivery by these devices. This explanation appears, for example, in "*Nicotine Addiction in Britain*[657] (p. 72)." The authors of this report, in appealing to this rescue hypothesis, ignore publications that did not find greater suppression of withdrawal symptoms with increased doses. They also took no notice of the absence of dose-response curves for suppression of withdrawal symptoms with these devices, or of the successful suppression of withdrawal symptoms with denicotized cigarettes.

An especially blatant example of ignoring powerful evidence against the hypothesis that nicotine is addictive is the inexplicable failure of smoking researchers to cite the numerous publications that did not find re-addiction to nicotine in ex-smokers who were exposed to nicotine transdermal patches for prolonged periods. One such study, referred to several times in this book[508], was published in the prominent and high-impact *New England Journal of Medicine*; yet, this study was cited in only two smoking related publications, versus in 139 studies on ulcerative colitis.

The view that nicotine is addicting, then, was successfully "enshrined" in the Surgeon General's Report. The resulting near-consensus in regard to this hypothesis and its complex social and political ramifications have created an atmosphere in which objective exploration of this hypothesis became practically impossible. Indeed, the possibility that nicotine may not be addictive has rarely been raised since 1988. The "enshrined" nicotine addiction has been uncritically adopted not only within the scientific community but also by the media; in fact, we have never heard a dissenting position expressed publicly. It is hardly surprising, therefore, that this view has had a profound effect on public beliefs regarding the nature of smoking. A 1977 study[159] reported that "*About four out of five non-smokers regarded the average cigarette smoker as an addict, whereas only about half the smokers saw themselves as addicted* (p.334)." In a study published eight years later[161], only 25 out of 2,312 subjects (1%) answered the question "How addicted do you think you are to smoking?" with the answer "Not at all." We would not be surprised if today, more than a decade after the Surgeon General published his report, it would turn out that both smokers and non-smokers view the statement "nicotine is addictive" as obviously true as "water is wet."

This, we submit, may be one of the worst effects of the nicotine addiction thesis. It most certainly managed to convince smokers that they are chemically addicted to smoking. As we have already mentioned in the introduction, perceptions and beliefs can have an critical effect on the success of quitting attempts. An addiction model inherently places control and responsibility outside the individual, so it is likely to undermine one's sense of control and self-efficacy. Indeed, smokers who believe that they are addicted perceive quitting as more difficult[321,334,407] and have reduced confidence in their ability to achieve complete cessation[160,161]. Moreover, these attitudes seem to act as self-fulfilling prophecies, as they are correlated with shorter duration of cessation attempts and higher relapse rates[470].

On a final note, we must stress that even if presenting smoking as nicotine addiction would have benefited the public, scientists should not be discouraged from opposing this thesis. The growth of knowledge depends on a continuous and unrelenting attitude of skepticism and a pluralism of opinions[365]. When views become "enshrined," whether or not this move is justified by the alleged welfare of the public, science is in danger of losing its edge over religion and propaganda. We believe that it is especially at such junctures that the critical attitude of scientists must be encouraged. We have already cited Cohen's exquisite explication of the devil's advocate's role in *"The dark side of religion*[107]" (see Chapter 1). We wish to add a related citation from the same article, with which we wholeheartedly identify (p. 294): *"I do not wish to suggest that I am merely an advocate, or that I have any doubts as to the justice of the arguments I have advanced. Doubtless some of my arguments may turn out to be erroneous, but at present I hold them all in good faith."* We hope that this book, even if some of its specific arguments turn out to be erroneous, will serve to "decanonize" and "disenshrine" the nicotine addiction hypothesis and to encourage an objective and critical re-evaluation of its scientific merits.

REFERENCES

1. Aarts, H., Paulussen, T., and Schaalma, H. (1997) Physical exercise habit: On the conceptualization and formation of habitual health behaviors. Health Education Research **12**:363-374.

2. Abelin, T., Buehler, A., Muller, P., Vesanen, K., and Imhof, P. R. (1989) Controlled trial of transdermal nicotine patch in tobacco withdrawal. Lancet **1**:7-10.

3. Acquas, E., Carboni, E., Leone, P., and Di Chiara, G. (1989) SCH23390 blocks drug-conditioned place-preference and place aversion:anhedonia (lack of reward) or apathy (lack of motivation) after dopamine-receptor blockade? Psychopharmacology **99**:151-155.

4. Acquas, E. and Di Chiara, G. (1992) Depression of mesolimbic dopamine transmission and sensitzation to morphine during opiate abstinence. J.Neurochem. **58**:1620-1625.

5. Adams, M. L. and Cicero, T. J. (1998) Nitric oxide mediates mecamylamine and naloxone-precipitated nicotine withdrawal. Eur.J.Pharmacol. **345**:R1-R2.

6. Adams, W. J., Lorens, S. A., and Mitchell, C. L. (1972) Morphine enhances lateral hypothalamic self-stimulation in the rat. Proc.Soc.Exp.Biol.Med. **140**:770-771.

7. Adlkofer, F., Scherer, G., Biber, A., Heller, W-D., and Lee, P. N. (1989) Consistency of nicotine intake in smokers of cigarettes with varying nicotine yields. In: Wald, N. and Froggatt, P. (*Eds.*): Nicotine, Smoking and the Low Tar Programme. Oxford University Press, Oxford.

8. Akers, R. L. (1991) Addiction: The troublesome concept. The Journal of Drug Issues **21**:777-793.

9. Allison, D. B., Fontaine, K. R., Manson, J. E., Stevens, J., and VanItallie, T. B. (1999) Annual deaths attributable to obesity in the United States. JAMA **282**:1530-1538.

10. American Psychiatric Association . (1994) Diagnostic and Statistical Manual of Mental Disorders, 4th Edition. Washington, DC.

11. Annau, Z. (1978) Electrical self-stimulation of the brain: A model for the behavioral evaluation of toxic agents. Environ.Health Perspect. **26**:59-67.

12. Aosaki, T., Graybiel, A. M., and Kimura, M. (1994) Effect of the nigrostriatal dopamine system on acquired neural responses in the striatum of behaving monkeys. Science **265**:412-415.

13. Aosaki, T., Kimura, M., and Graybiel, A. M. (1995) Temporal and spatial characteristics of tonically active neurons of the primate's striatum. J.Neurophysiol. **73**:1234-1252.

14. Apel, M., Klein, K., McDermott, R. J., and Westhoff, W. W. (1997) Restricting smoking at the University of Koln, Germany – a case study. J.Am.College.Hlth. **45**:219-223.

15. Aravich, P. F., Stanley, E. Z., and Doerries, L. E. (1985) Exercise in food-restricted rats produces 2DG feeding and metabolic abnormalities similar to anorexia nervosa. Physiol.Behav. **57**:147-153.

16. Arnold, B. K., Allison, S. I., Paetsch, T. P., and Greenshaw, A. J. (1995) 5HT3 receptor antagonists do not block nicotine induced hyperactivity in rats. Psychopharmacology **119**:213-221.

17. Arregui-Aguirre, A., Claro-Izaguirre, F., Goni-Garrido, M. J., Zarate-Oleaga, J. A., and Morgado-Bernal, I. (1987) Effects of acute nicotine and ethanol on medial prefrontal cortex self-stimulation in rats. Pharmacol.Biochem.Behav. **27**:15-20.

18. Asch, S. E. (1958) Effects of group pressure upon modification and distortion of judgements. In: Maccoby, E. E., Newcomb, T. M., and Hartley, E. L. (*Eds.*): Readings in Social Psychology. Rigehart and Winston, New York.

19. Ashton, H. and Stepney, R. (1982) Smoking psychology and pharmacology. Travistock Publications, London.

20. Ashton, H. and Watson, D. W. (1970) Puffing frequency and nicotine intake in cigarette smokers. Br.Med.J. **3**:679-681.

21. Ator, N. A. and Griffiths, R. R. (1983) Nicotine self-administration in baboons. Pharmacol.Biochem.Behav. **19**:993-1003.

22. Atrens, D. M. and Becker, F. T. (1975) Assessing the aversiveness of intracranial self-stimulation. Psychopharmacologia **44**:159-163.

23. Atrens, D. M., Becker, F. T., and Hunt, G. E. (1980) Apomorphine: selective inhibition of the aversive component of lateral hypothalamic self-stimulation. Psychopharmacology 71:97-99.

24. Atrens, D. M., Williams, M. P., Brady, C. J., and Hunt, G. E. (1982) Energy balance and hypothalamic self-stimulation. Behav.Brain Res. 5:131-142.

25. Baldinger, B., Hasenfratz, M., and Battig, K. (1995) Effects of smoking abstinence and nicotine abstinence on heart rate, activity and cigarette craving under field conditions. Psychopharmacology 10:127-136.

26. Baldinger, B., Hasenfratz, M., and Battig, K. (1995) Switching to ultralow nicotine cigarettes: Effects of different tar yields and blocking of olfactory cues. Pharmacol.Biochem.Behav. 50:233-239.

27. Balfour, D. J. K. (1990) A comparison of the effects of nicotine and (+)-amphetamine on rat behavior in an unsignalled Sidman avoidance schedule. J.Pharm.Pharmacol. 42:257-260.

28. Balleine, B. W. (1991) The acquisition of self-stimulation of the medial prefrontal cortex following exposure to escapable or inescapable footshock. Behav.Brain Res. 43:167-174.

29. Baltzer, J. H., Levitt, R. A., and Furby, J. E. (1977) Etorphine and shuttle-box self-stimulation in the rat. Pharmacol.Biochem.Behav. 7:413-416.

30. Bandura, A., Adams, N. E., Hardy, A. B., and Howells, G. N. (1980) Tests of the generality of self-efficacy theory. Cognit.Ther.Res. 4:39-66.

31. Bardo, M. T., Green, T. A., Crooks, P. A., and Dwoskin, L. P. (1999) Nornicotine is self-administered intravenously by rats. Psychopharmacology 146:290-296.

32. Bardo, M. T., Valone, J. M., and Bevins, R. A. (1999) Locomotion and conditioned place preference produced by acute intravenous amphetamine: Role of dopamine receptors and individual differences in amphetamine self-administration. Psychopharmacology 143:39-46.

33. Barjavel, M. J., Scherrmann, J. M., and Bhargava, H. N. (1995) Relationship between morphine analgesia and cortical extracellular fluid levels of morphine and its metabolites in the rat: A microdialysis study. Br.J.Pharmac. 116:3205-3210.

34. Barrass, B. C., Blackburn, J. W., Brimblecombe, R. W., and Rich, P. (1969) Modification of nicotine toxicity by pretreatment with different drugs. Biomed.Pharmacol. 18:2145-2152.

35. Battig, K., Driscoll, P., Schlatter, J., and Uster, H. J. (1976) Effects of nicotine on the exploratory locomotion patterns of female Roman high- and low-avoidance rats. Pharmacol.Biochem.Behav. 4:435-439.

36. Bauco, P., Wang, Y., and Wise, R. A. (1993) Lack of sensitization or tolerance to the facilitating effect of ventral tegmental area morphine on lateral hypothalamic brain stimulation reward. Brain Res. **617**:303-308.

37. Bauco, P. and Wise, R. A. (1994) Potentiation of lateral hypothalamic and midline mesencephalic brain stimulation reinforcement by nicotine: examination of repeated treatment. J.Pharmacol.exp.Ther. **271**:294-301.

38. Baumeister, A. A., Anticich, T. G., Hebert, G., Hawkins, M. F., and Nagy, M. (1989) Evidence that physical dependence on morphine is mediated by the ventral midbrain. Neuropharmacol. **28**:1151-1157.

39. Bechara, A. and Van der Kooy, D. (1992) Lesions of the tegmental pedunculopontine nucleus: Effects on the locomotor activity induced by morphine and amphetamine. Pharmacol.Biochem.Behav. **42**:9-18.

40. Behm, F. M., Schur, C., Levin, E. D., Tashkin, D. P., and Rose, J. E. (1993) Clinical evaluation of a citric inhaler for smoking cessation. Drug Alc.Depend. **31**:131-138.

41. Beninger, R. J. (1983) The role of dopamine in locomotor activity and learning. Brain Res. **287**:173-196.

42. Benowitz, N. L. (1996) Pharmacology of nicotine: addiction and therapeutics. Ann.Rev.Pharmacol.Toxicol. **36**:597-613.

43. Benowitz, N. L. (1999) Nicotine addiction. Prim.Care **26**:611-631.

44. Benowitz, N. L., Hall, S. M., Herning, R. I., Jacob, P. I., Jones, R. T., and Osman, A. L. (1983) Smokers of low-yield cigarettes do not consume less nicotine. N.England J.Med. **309**:139-142.

45. Benowitz, N. L. and Jacob, P. (1990) Intravenous nicotine replacement suppresses nicotine intake from cigarette smoking. J.Pharmacol.exp.Ther. **254**:1000-1005.

46. Benowitz, N. L., Jacob, P., Jones, R. T., and Rosenberg, J. (1982) Interindividual variability in the metabolism and cardiovascular effects of nicotine in man. J.Pharmacol.exp.Ther. **221**:368-372.

47. Benowitz, N. L., Jacob, P. I., Yu, L., Talcott, R., Hall, S., and Jones, R. T. (1986) Reduced tar, nicotine, and carbon monoxide exposure with smoking ultralow- but not low-yield cigarettes. JAMA **256**:241-246.

48. Benowitz, N. L., Kuyt, F., and Jacob, O. III. (1982) Circadian blood nicotine concentrations during cigarette smoking. Clin.Pharmacol.Ther. **32** :758-764.

49. Benowitz, N. L., Zevin, S., and Jacob, P. (1998) Suppression of nicotine intake during ad libitum cigarette smoking by high-dose transdermal nicotine. J.Pharmacol.exp.Ther. **287**:958-962.

50. Berridge, K. C. and Robinson, T. E. (1998) What is the role of dopamine in reward: Hedonic impact, reward leraning, or incentive salience? Brain Res.Rev. **28**:309-369.

51. Berridge, V. and Edwards, G. (1987) Opium and the People: Opiate Use in Nineteenth-Century England. Yale University, New Haven, CT.

52. Bhargava, H. N., Villar, V. M., Rahmani, N. H., and Larsen, A. K. (1992) Studies on the possible role of pharmacokinetics in the development of tolerance to morphine in the rat . Gen.Pharmacol. **6**:1199-1204.

53. Biener, L., Cullen, D., Di, Z. X., and Hammond, S. K. (1997) Household smoking restrictions and adolescents exposure to environmental tobacco-smoke. Prevent. Med. **26**:358-363.

54. Bjornson-Benson, W., Nides, M., Dolce, J., Rand, C., Lindgren, P., O'Hara, P., and Buist, A. S. (1993) Nicotine use in the first years of the Lung Health Study. Addict.Behav. **18**:491-502.

55. Black, D. W. (1998) Recognition and treatment of obsessive-compulsive spectrum disorders . In: Swinson, R. P. et al. (*Eds.*): Obsessive-Compulsive Disorder: Theory, Research, and Treatment. Guilford, New York.

56. Blass, E. M. and Ciaramitaro, V. (1994) A new look at some old mechanisms in human newborns: Taste and tactile determinants of state, affect, and action. Monographs of the Society for Research in Child Development **59**:v81.

57. Boren, J. J., Stitzner, M. L., and Henningfield, J. E. (1990) Preference among research cigarettes with varying nicotine yields. Pharmacol.Biochem.Behav. **36**:191-193.

58. Bozarth, M. A., Pudiak, C. M., and KuoLee, R. (1998) Effect of chronic nicotine on brain stimulation reward. I. Effect of daily injections. Behav.Brain Res. **96**:185-188.

59. Bozarth, M. A., Pudiak, C. M., and KuoLee, R. (1998) Effect of chronic nicotine on brain stimulation reward. II. An escalating regimen. Behav.Brain Res. **96**:189-194.

60. Bozarth, M. A. and Wise, R. A. (1985) Toxicity associated with long-term intravenous heroin and cocaine self-administration in the rat. JAMA **254**:81-83.

61. Brauer, L. H., Behm, F. M., Westman, P. P., and Rose, J. E. (1999) Naltrexone blockade of nicotine effects in cigarette smokers. Psychopharmacology **143**:339-346.

62. Brecher, E. M. (1972) Licit and Illicit Drugs. Little, Brown and Company, Boston.

63. Brenner, H., Born, J., Novak, P., and Wanek, V. (1997) Smoking-behavior and attitude toward smoking regulations and passive smoking in the workplace – a study among 974 employees in the German metal-industry. Prevent.Med. **26**:138-143.

64. Brenner, H. and Fleischle, B. (1994) Smoking regulations at the workplace and smoking-behavior – a study from Southern Germany. Prevent.Med. **23**:230-234.

65. Bridges, R. B., Combs, J. G., Humble, J. W., Turbek, J. A., Rehm, S. R., and Haley, N. J. (1990) Population characteristics and cigarette yield as determinants of smoke exposure. Pharmacol.Biochem.Behav. **37**:17-28.

66. Bridges, R. B., Humble, J. W., Turbek, J. A., and Rehm, S. R. (1986) Smoking history, cigarette yield and smoking behavior as determinants of smoke exposure. Eur.J.Respir.Dis. **69(Suppl.146)**:129-137.

67. Brigham, J., Gross, J., Stitzer, M. L., and Felch, L. J. (1994) Effects of restricted work-site smoking policy on employees who smoke. Am.J.Pub.Health **84**:773-778.

68. Brioni, J. D., Kim, D. J. B., O'Neill, A. B., Williams, J. E. G., and Decker, M. W. (1994) Clozapine attenuates the discriminative stimulus properties of (-)-nicotine. Brain Res. **643**:1-9.

69. Brodie, D. A., Moreno, O. M., Malis, J. L., and Boren, J. J. (1960) Rewarding properties of intracranial stimulation. Science **131**:929-930.

70. Brown, E. E. and Fibiger, H. C. (1993) Differential effects of exitotoxic lesions of the amygdala on cocaine-induced conditioned locomotion and conditioned place preference. Psychopharmacology **113**:123-130.

71. Browne, R. G. and Segal, D. S. (1980) Behavioral activating effects of opiates and opioid peptides. Biol.Psychiat. **15**:77-86.

72. Bush, H. D., Bush, M. F., Miller, M. A., and Reid, L. D. (1976) Addictive agents and intracranial stimulation: Daily morphine and lateral hypothalamic self-stimulation. Physiol.Psychol. **4**:79-85.

73. Butschky, M. F., Bailey, D., and Henningfield, J. E. (1995) Smoking without nicotine delivery decreases withdrawal in 12-hour abstinent smokers. Pharmacol.Biochem.Behav. **50**:91-96.

74. Cabeza De Vaca, S., Holiman, S., and Carr, K. D. (1998) A search for the metabolic signal that sensitizes lateral hypothalamic self-stimulation in food-restricted rats. Physiol.Behav. **64**:251-260.

75. Caggiula, A. R. and Hoebel, B. G. (1966) "Copulation-Reward Site" in the posterior hypothalamus. Science **153**:1284-1285.

76. Cain, W. S. (1980) Sensory attributes of cigarette smoking. In: Gori, G. B. and Bock, F. G. (*Eds.*): Banbury Report 3: A Safe Cigarette? Cold Spring Laboratory, New York.

77. Calabresi, P., Lacey, M. G., and North, R. A. (1989) Nicotine excitation of rat ventral tegmental neurones in vitro studied by intracellular recording. Br.J.Pharmacol. **98**:135-140.

78. Calcagnetti, D. J. and Schechter, M. D. (1994) Nicotine place preference using the biased method of conditioning. Prog.Neuropsychopharmacol.Biol.Psychiat. **18**:925-933.

79. Campbell, I. A., Prescott, R. J., and Tjeder-Burton, S. M. (1996) Transdermal nicotine plus support in patients attending hospital with smoking-related diseases: A placebo-controlled study. Respir.Med. **90**:47-51.

80. Campos, R. G. (1989) Soothing pain-elicited distress in infants with swaddling and pacifiers. Child Dev. **60**:781-792.

81. Campos, R. G. (1994) Rocking and pacifiers: Two comforting interventions for heelstick pain. Res.Nurs.Hlth. **17**:321-331.

82. Carboni, E. E., Acquas, P. L., and Di Chiara, G. (1989) 5HT3 receptor antagonists block morphine and nicotine – but not amphetamine-induced reward. Psychopharmacology **97**:175-178.

83. Carlezon, W. A., Jr. and Wise, R. A. (1993) Morphine-induced potentiation of brain stimulation reward is enhanced by MK-801. Brain Res. **620**:339-342.

84. Carrera, M. R., Schulteis, G., and Koob, G. F. (1999) Heroin self-administration in dependent Wistar rats: Increased sensitivity to naloxone. Psychopharmacology **144**:111-120.

85. Carroll, M. E., Lac, S. T., Asencio, M., and Keenan, R. M. (1989) Nicotine dependence in rats. Life Sci. **45**:1381-1388.

86. Castellani, B. and Rugle, L. (1995) A comparison of pathological gamblers to alcoholics and cocaine misusers on impulsivity, sensation seeking, and craving. Int.J.Addict. **30**:275-289.

87. Castellanos, F. X., Ritchie, G. F., Marsh, W. L., and Rappoport, J. L. (1996) DSM-IV stereotypic movement disorder: Persistence of stereotypies of infancy in intellectually normal adolescents and adults. J.Clin.Psychiatry **57**:116-122.

88. Catania, H. (1998) Medical co-prescription of heroin to heroin addicts: State of the art and future directions. Conference Transcript, Utrecht.

89. Cepeda-Benito, A. (1993) Meta-analytical review of the efficacy of nicotine chewing gum in smoking treatment programs. J.Cons.Clin.Psychol. **61**:822-830.

90. Chance, W. T., Murfin, D., Krynock, G. M., and Rosecrans, J. A. (1977) A description of the nicotine stimulus and tests of its generalization to amphetamine. Psychopharmacology **55**:19-26.

91. Chapman, S., Borland, R., Scollo, M., Brownson, R. C., Dominello, A., and Woodward, S. (1999) The impact of smoke-free workplaces on declining cigarette consumption in Australia and the United States. Am.J.Pub.Hlth **89**:1018-1023.

92. Cherry, W. H. and Forbes, W. F. (1972) Canadian studies aimed toward a less harmful cigarette. J.Natl.Cancer Inst. **48**:1765-1773.

93. Chesnokova, V., Auernhammer, C. J., and Melmed, S. (1998) Murine leukemia inhibitory factor gene disruption attenuates the hypothalamo-pituitary-adrenal axis stress response. Endocrinology **139**:2209-2216.

94. Chiamulera, C., Borgo, C., Falchetto, S., Valerio, E., and Tessari, M. (1996) Nicotine reinstatement of nicotine self-administration after long-term extinction. Psychopharmacology **127**:102-107.

95. Chinen, C. C. and Frussa-Filho, R. (1999) Conditioning to injection procedures and repeated testing increase SCH 23390-induced catalepsy in mice. Neuropsychopharmacol. **21**:670-678.

96. Cinciripini, P. M., Ciniciripini, L. G., Wallfish, A., Haque, W., and Vanvunakis, H. (1996) Behavioral-Therapy and the transdermal nicotine patch – effects on cessation outcome. J.Cons.Clin.Psychol. **64**:314-323.

97. Clarke, P. B. and Fibiger, H. C. (1987) Apparent absence of nicotine-induced conditioned place preference in rats. Psychopharmacology **92**:84-88.

98. Clarke, P. B., Fu, D. S., Jakubovic, A., and Fibiger, H. C. (1988) Evidence that mesolimbic dopaminergic activation underlies the locomotor stimulant action of nicotine in rats . J.Pharmacol.exp.Ther. **246**:701-708.

99. Clarke, P. B. and Kumar, R. (1983) Characterization of the locomotor stimulant action of nicotine in tolerant rats. Br.J.Pharmacol. **80**:587-594.

100. Clarke, P. B. and Kumar, R. (1984) Effects of nicotine and d-amphetamine on intracranial self-stimulation in a shuttle box test in rats. Psychopharmacology **84**:109-114.

101. Clarke, P. B. S. and Kumar, R. (1983) Nicotine does not improve discrimination of brain stimulation reward by rats. Psychopharmacology **79**:271-277.

102. Clarke, P. B. S. and Kumar, R. (1983) The effects of nicotine on locomotor activity in non-tolerant and tolerant rats. Br.J.Pharmac. **78**:329-337.

103. Clarke, P. B. S. and Kumar, R. (1984) Some effects of nicotine on food and water intake in underprived rats. Br.J.Pharmac. **82**:233-239.

104. Clausen, J. A. (1977) Early history of narcotics use and narcotics legislation in the United States. In: Rock, P. E. (*Ed.*): Drugs and Politics. Transaction Books, New Brunswick, N.J.

105. Cohen, J. D. and Servan-Schreiber, D. (1993) A theory of dopamine function and its role in cognitive deficits in schizophrenia. Schizophren.Bull. **19**:85-104.

106. Cohen, L. M., Collins, J. F. L., and Britt, D. M. (1997) The effect of chewing gum on tobacco withdrawal. Addict.Behav. **22**:769-773.

107. Cohen, M. R. (1964) The dark side of religion. In: Kaufman, W. (*Ed.*): Religion from Tolstoy to Camus. Harper & Row, New York.

108. Cohen, S., Lichtenstein, E., Porochaska, J. O., Rossi, J. S., Gritz, E. R., Carr, C. R., Orleans, C. T., Schoenbach, V. J., Biener, L., Abrams, D., DiClemente, C., Curry, S., Marlatt, G. A., Cummings, K. M., Emont, S. L., Giovini, G., and Ossip-Klein, D. (1989) Debunking myths about self-quitting . Evidence from 10 prospective studies of persons who attempt to quit smoking by themselves. Am.Psychologist **44**:1355-1365.

109. Conze, C., Scherer, G., Tricker, A. R., and Adlkofer, F. (1994) The influence of orally resorbed nicotine on smoking behavior. Presented at the International Symposium of Nicotine: The Effects of Nicotine on Biological Systems II. Montreal, July 1994. C.f. Pritchard et al., 1996.

110. Conze, C., Scherer, G., Tricker, A. R., and Adlkofer, F. (1995) The influence of orally resorbed nicotine on smoking behaviour. 1st Annual Scientific Conference of the Society for Research on Nicotine and Tobacco (SRNT), March 24-25, 1995, San Diego, USA.

111. Coons, E. E. and Cruce, J. A. F. (1968) Lateral hypothalamus: Food, current intensity in maintaining self-stimulation of hunger. Science **159**:1117-1119.

112. Copeland, R. L. and Pradhan, S. N. (1988) Effect of morphine on self-stimulation in rats and its modification by chloramphenicol. Pharmacol. Biochem.Behav. **31**:933-935.

113. Corbett, D. (1992) Chronic morphine fails to enhance the reward value of prefrontal cortex self-stimulation. Pharmacol.Biochem.Behav. **42**:451-455.

114. Cordova, C. R. J. (1988) Smoking Cessation in a Cohort of Smokers using different self-help guides.

115. Corrigall, W. A. and Coen, K. M. (1989) Nicotine maintains robust self-administration in rats on a limited-access schedule. Psychopharmacology **99**:473-478.

116. Corrigall, W. A. and Coen, K. M. (1991) Opiate antagonists reduce cocaine but not nicotine self-administration. Psychopharmacology **104**:167-170.

117. Corrigall, W. A. and Coen, K. M. (1991) Selective dopamine antagonists reduce nicotine self-administration. Psychopharmacology **104**:171-176.

118. Corrigall, W. A. and Coen, K. M. (1994) Nicotine self-administration and locomotor activity are not modified by the 5-HT3 antagonists ICS 205-930 and MDL 72222. Pharmacol.Biochem.Behav. **49**:67-71.

119. Corrigall, W. A., Coen, K. M., and Adamson, K. L. (8-8-1994) Self-administered nicotine activates the mesolimbic dopamine system through the ventral tegmental area. Brain Res. **653**:278-284.

120. Corrigall, W. A., Franklin, K. B., Coen, K. M., and Clarke, P. B. (1992) The mesolimbic dopaminergic system is implicated in the reinforcing effects of nicotine. Psychopharmacology **107**:285-289.

121. Corrigall, W. A., Herling, S., and Coen, K. M. (1989) Evidence for a behavioral deficit during withdrawal from chronic nicotine treatment. Pharmacol. Biochem.Behav. **33**:559-562.

122. Cox, B. M., Goldstein, A., and Nelson, W. T. (1984) Nicotine self- administration in rats. Br.J.Pharmacol. **83**:49-55.

123. Creighton, D. E. and Lewis, P. H. (1978) The effect of different cigarettes on human smoking patterns. In: Thornton, R. E. (*Ed.*): Smoking Behaviour. Churhill Livingstone, Edinburgh.

124. Cummings, K. M., Hyland, A, Ockene, J. K., Hymowitz, N., and Manley, M. (1997) Use of the nicotine skin patch by smokers in 20 communities in the United States, 1992-1993. Tobacco Control **6(Suppl 2)**:S63-S70.

125. Cunningham, C. L. (1979) Flavor and location aversions produced by ethanol. Behav.Neural Biol. **27**:362-367.

126. Cunningham, C. L., Mallott, D. H., Dickenson, S. D., and Risinger, F. O. (1992) Haloperidol does not alter expression of ethanol-induced conditioned place preference. Behav.Brain Res. **50**:1-5.

127. D'Angio, M. B., Serrano, A., Rivy, J. P., and Scatton, B. (1987) Tail pinch stress increases extracellular DOPAC levels (as measured by in vivo voltammetry) in rat nucleus accumbens but not frontal cortex: Antagonism by diazepam and zolpidem. Brain Res. **409**:169-174.

128. D'Angio, M. B., Serrano, A., Scatton, B., and Scatton, J. P. (1990) Mesocorticolimbic dopaminergic systems and emotional states. J.Neurosci.Meth. **34**:135-142.

129. Dai, S., Corrigall, W. A., Coen, K. M., and Kalant, H. (1989) Heroin self-administration by rats: Influence of dose and physical dependence. Pharmacol.Biochem.Behav. **32**:1009-1015.

130. Dale, L. C., Hurt, R. D., Offord, K. P., Lawson, G. M., Croghan, I. T., and Schroeder, D. R. (1995) High-dose nicotine patch therapy. Percentage of replacement and smoking cessation. JAMA **274**:1353-1358.

131. Danaher, B. G. (1977) Research on rapid smoking: Interim summary and recommendations. Addict.Behav. **2**:151-166.

132. Daughton, D. M., Heatley, S. A., Prendergast, J. J., Causey, D., Knowles, M., Rolf, C. N., Cheney, R. A., Hatlelid, K., Thompson, A. B., and Rennard, S. I. (1991) Effect of transdermal nicotine delivery as an adjunct to low-intervention smoking cessation therapy. Arch.Intern.Med. **151**:749-752.

133. Davis, C. (1997) Eating disorders and hyperactivity: A psychobiological perspective. Can.J.Psychiatry **42**:168-175.

134. Davis, C. and Claridge, G. (1998) The eating disorders as addiction: A psychobiological perspective. Addict.Behav. **23**:463-475.

135. Davis, C., Kennedy, S. H., Ravelski, E., and Dionne, M. (1994) The role of physical activity in the development and maintenance of eating disorders. Psychol.Med. **24**:957-967.

136. De La Garza, R. and Johanson, C. E. (1987) The effects of food deprivation on the self-administration of psychoactive drugs. Drug Alc.Depend. **19**:17-27.

137. Deakin, J. F. (1980) On the neurochemical basis of self-stimulation with midbrain raphe electrode placements. Pharmacol.Biochem.Behav. **13**:525-530.

138. Dessirier, J., O'Mahony, M., and Carstens, E. (1997) Oral irritant effects of nicotine: Psychophysical evidence for decreased sensation following repeated application and lack of cross-sensitization to capsaicin. Chem.Senses **22**:483-492.

139. Dessirier, J., O'Mahony, M., Sieffermann, J., and Carstens, E. (1998) Mecamylamine inhibits nicotine but not capsaicin irritation on the tongue: Psychophysical evidence that nicotine and capsaicin activate separate molecular receptors. Neurosci.Lett. **240**:65-68.

140. Deutsch, J. A. and DiCara, L. (1967) Hunger and extinction in intracranial self-stimulation. J.Comp.Physiol.Psychol. **63**:344-347.

141. Deutsch, J. A. and Howarth, C. I. (1962) Evocation by fear of a habit learned for electrical stimulation of the brain. Science **136**:1057-1058.

142. Deutsch, J. A. and Howarth, C. I. (1963) Some tests of a theory of intracranial self-stimulation. Psychol.Rev. **70**:444-460.

143. DiChiara, G. (1998) A motivational learning hypothesis of the role of mesolimbic dopamine in compulsive drug use. J.Psychopharmacol. **12**:54-67.

144. Djordjevic, M. V., Fan, J., Ferguson, S., and Hoffmann, D. (1995) Self-regulation of smoking intensity. Smoke yields of the low-nicotine, low-tar cigarettes. Carcinogenesis **16**:2015-2021.

145. Doherty, K., Kinnunen, T., Militello, F. S., and Garvey, A. J. (1995) Urges to smoke during the first month of abstinence: Relationship to relapse and predictors. Psychopharmacology **119**:171-178.

146. Domjan, M. and Burkhard, B. (1986) The Principles of Learning and Behavior. Brooks/Cole Publishing Company, Monterey, CA.

147. Donny, E. C., Caggiula, A. R., Knopf, S., and Brown, C. (1995) Nicotine self-administration in rats. Psychopharmacology **122**:390-394.

148. Donny, E. C., Caggiula, A. R., Mielke, M. M., Jacobs, K. S., Rose, C., and Sved, A. F. (1998) Acquisition of nicotine self-administration in rats: The effects of dose, feeding schedule, and drug contingency. Psychopharmacology **136**:83-90.

149. Dougherty, J., Miller, D., Todd, G., and Kostenbauder, H. B. (1981) Reinforcing and other behavioral effects of nicotine. Neurosci.Biobehav.Rev. **5**:487-495.

150. Driessen, F. M. H. M. (1990) Methadoneverstrekking in Nederland. Bureau Driessen Sociaal Wetenschappelijk Onderzoek en Advies, Rijswijk/Utrecht.

151. Druhan, J. P., Fibiger, H. C., and Phillips, A. G. (1989) Differential effects of cholinergic drugs on discriminative cues and self-stimulation produced by electrical stimulation of the ventral tegmental area. Psychopharmacology **97**:331-338.

152. Dunn, P. J. and Freiesleben, E. R. (1978) The effects of nicotine-enhanced cigarettes on human smoking parameters and aveolar carbon monoxide levels. In: Thornton, R. E. (*Ed.*): Smoking Behaviour. Churchill Livingstone, New York.

153. Dwoskin, L. P., Crooks, P. A., Teng, L., Green, T. A., and Bardo, M. T. (1999) Acute and chronic effects on locomotor activity in rats: Altered response to nicotine. Psychopharmacology **145**:442-451.

154. Ebert, R. V., McNabb, M. E., McCuster, K. T., and Snow, S. L. (1983) Amount of nicotine and carbon monoxide inhaled by smokers of low-tar, low-nicotine cigarettes. JAMA **250**:2840-2842.

155. Ebert, R. V., McNabb, M. E., McCuster, K. T., and Snow, S. L. (1984) Effect of nicotine chewing gum on plasma nicotine levels of cigarette smokers. Clin.Pharmacol.Ther. **35**:495-498.

156. Eddy, N. B., Halbach, H., Isbell, H., and Seevers, M. (1965) Drug dependence: Its significance and characteristics. Bulletin of the World Health Organization **32**:721-733.

157. Edmonds, D. E., Stellar, J. R., and Gallistel, C. R. (1974) Parametric analysis of brain stimulation reward in the rat: II. Temporal summation in the reward system. J.Comp.Physiol.Psychol. **87**:869.

158. Eisen, J. L., Goodman, W. K., Keller, M. B., Warshaw, M. G., De Marco, M. S. P. H., Luce, D. D., and Rasmussen, S. A. (1999) Patterns of remission and relapse in obsessive-compulsive disorder: A 2-year prospective study. J.Clin.Psychiatry **60**:346-351.

159. Eiser, J. R., Sutton, S. R., and Wober, M. (1977) Smokers, non-smokers and the attribution of addiction. Br.J.soc.clin.Psychol. **16**:329-336.

160. Eiser, J. R. and van der Pligt, J. (1986) Smoking cessation and smokers' perceptions of their addiction. J.Soc.Clin.Psychol. **4**:60-70.

161. Eiser, J. R., van der Pligt, J., Raw, M., and Sutton, S. R. (1985) Trying to stop smoking: Effects of perceived addiction, attributions for failure, and expectancy of success. J.Behav.Med. **8**:321-341.

162. Eissenberg, T., Griffiths, R. R., and Stitzer, M. L. (1996) Mecamylamine does not precipitate withdrawal in cigarette smokers. Psychopharmacology **127**:328- 336.

163. Elder, S. T., Montgomery, N. P., and Rye, M. M. (1965) Effects of food deprivation and methamphetamine on fixed-ratio schedules of intracranial self-stimulation. Psychol.Rep. **16**:1225-1237.

164. Epping-Jordan, M. P., Watkins, S. S., Koob, G. F., and Markou, A. (1998) Dramatic decreases in brain reward function during nicotine withdrawal. Nature **393**:76-79.

165. Ernster, V. L., Grady, D. G., Greene, J. C., Walsh, M., Robertson, P., Daniels, T. E., Benowitz, N. L., Siegel, D., Gerbert, B., and Hauck, W. W. (1990) Smokeless tobacco use and health effects among baseball players. JAMA **264**: 218-224.

166. Esposito, R. and Kornetsky, C. (1977) Morphine lowering of self-stimulation thresholds: Lack of tolerance with long-term administration. Science **195**:189- 191.

167. Esposito, R. U. and Kornetsky, C. (1978) Opioids and rewarding brain stimulation. Neurosci.Biobehav.Rev. **2**:115-122.

168. Esposito, R. U., McLean, S., and Kornetsky, C. (1977) Effects of morphine on intracranial self-stimulation to various brain stem loci. Brain Res. **168**:425-429.

169. Ettenberg, A., Petit, H. O., Bloom, F. E., and Koob, G. F. (1982) Heroin and cocaine intravenous self-administration in rats: Mediation by separate neural systems. Psychopharmacology **78**:204-209.

170. Fagerstrom, K. O. (1982) Effects of a nicotine-enriched cigarette on nicotine titration, daily cigarette consumption, and levels of carbon monoxide, cotinine, and nicotine. Psychopharmacology **77**:164-167.

171. Farkas, A. J., Gilpin, E. A., Distefan, J. M., and Pierce, J. P. (1999) The effects of household and workplace smoking restrictions on quitting behaviors. Tobacco Control **8**:261-265.

172. Farrelly, M. C., Evans, W. N., and Sfekas, A. E. (1999) The impact of workplace smoking bans: Results from a national survey. Tobacco Control **8**:272-277.

173. Ferrari, C. M., O'Connor, D. A., and Riley, A. L. (1991) Cocaine-induced taste aversions: Effect of route of administration. Pharmacol.Biochem.Behav. **38**:267-271.

174. Fiore, M. C., Jorenby, D. E., Baker, T. B., and Kenford, S. L. (1992) Tobacco dependence and the nicotine patch. Clinical guidelines for effective use. JAMA **268**:2687-2694.

175. Fiore, M. C., Kenford, S. L., Jorenby, D. E., Wetter, D. W., Smith, S. S., and Baker, T. B. (1994) 2 Studies of the clinical effectiveness of the nicotine patch with different counseling treatments. Chest **105**:524-533.

176. Fiore, M. E., Smith, S. S., Jorenby, D. E., and Baker, T. B. (1994) The effectiveness of the nicotine patch for smoking cessation: A meta-analysis. JAMA **271**:1940-1947.

177. Fischer, J. L., Pidoplichko, V. I., and Dani, J. A. (1998) Nicotine modifies the activity of ventral tegmental area dopaminergic neurons and hippocampal GABAergic neurons. J.Physiol.(Paris) **92**:209-213.

178. Flaten, M. A. and Blumenthal, T. D. (1999) Caffeine-associated stimuli elicit conditioned responses: An experimental model of the placebo effect. Psychopharmacology **145**:105-112.

179. Flegal, M. D., Carroll, R. J., Kuczmarski, R. J., and Johnson, C. L. (1998) Overweight and obesity in the United States: Prevalence and trends. Int.J.Obes. Relat.Metab.Disord. **22**:39-47.

180. Flynn, F. W., Webster, M., and Ksir, C. (1989) Chronic voluntary nicotine drinking enhances nicotine palatablility. Behav.Neurosci. **103**:356-364.

181. Forbes, W. F., Robinson, J. C., Hanley, J. A., and Colburn, H. N. (1976) Studies on the nicotine exposure of individual smokers. 1. Changes in the mouth-level exposure to nicotine on switching to lower nicotine cigarettes. Int.J.Addict. **11**:933-950.

182. Ford, R. D. and Balster, R. L. (1976) Schedule-controlled behavior in the morphine-dependent rat. Pharmacol.Biochem.Behav. **4**:569-573.

183. Foulds, J., McSorley, K., Sneddon, J., Feyerabend, C., Jarvis, M. J., and Russell, M. A. H. (1994) Effects of subcutaneous nicotine injections on EEG alpha frequency in non-smokers: A placebo-controlled pilot study. Psycho- pharmacology **115**:163-166.

184. Foulds, J., Stapleton, J., Bell, N., Swettenham, J., Jarvis, M. J., and Russell, M. A. H. (1997) Mood and physiological effects of subcutaneous nicotine in smokers and never-smokers. Drug Alc.Depend. **44**:105-115.

185. Foulds, J., Stapleton, J., Feyerabend, C., Vesey, C., Jarvis, M. J., and Russell, M. A. H. (1992) Effects of transdermal nicotine patches on cigarette smoking: A double blind crossover study. Psychopharmacology **106**:421-427.

186. Fouriezos, G., Hansson, P., and Wise, R. A. (1978) Neuroleptic-induced attenuation of brain stimulation reward in rats. J.Comp.Physiol.Psychol. **92**:661- 671.

187. Fouriezos, G. and Wise, R. A. (1976) Pimozide-induced extinction of intracranial self-stimulation: Response patterns rule out motor or performance deficits. Brain Res. **103**:377-380.

188. Fox, A. and Schaefer, C. (1996) Pacifier use in young children: Practical research findings. Psychology: A Journal of Human Behavior **33**:30-34.

189. Friedman, I., Dar, R., and Shilony, E. (2000) Compulsivity and obsessionality in opioid addiction. J.Nerv.Mental Disease **188**:155-162.

190. Friedman, S. and Fletcher, C. M. (1976) Changing in smoking habits and cough in men smoking cigarettes with 30% NSM tobacco substitute. Br.Med.J. **1**:1427-1430.

191. Frith, C. D. (1971) The effect of varying the nicotine of cigarettes on human smoking behavior. Psychopharmacologia **19**:188-192.

192. Frost, C., Fullerton, F. M., Stephen, A. M., Stone, R., Nicolaides-Bouman, A., Densem, J., Wald, N. J., and Semmence, A. (1995) The tar reduction study: Randomised trial of the effect of cigarette tar yield reduction on compensatory smoking. Thorax **50**:1038-1043.

193. Frutiger, S. A. (1986) Changes in self-stimulation at stimulation-bound eating and drinking sites in the lateral hypothalamus during food or water deprivation, glucoprivation, and intracellular or extracellular dehydration. Behav.Neurosci. **100**:221-229.

194. Fudala, P. J. and Iwamoto, E. T. (1986) Further studies on nicotine-induced conditioned place preference in the rat. Pharmacol.Biochem.Behav. **25**:1041-1049.

195. Fudala, P. J., Iwamoto, E. T., and Teoh, K. W. (1985) Pharmacologic characterization of nicotine-induced conditioned place preference. Pharmacol. Biochem.Behav. **22**:237-241.

196. Fung, Y. K. (1990) The importance of the nucleus accumbens in nicotine- induced locomotor activity. J.Pharm.Pharmacol. **42**:595-596.

197. Gallistel, C. R. (1966) Motivating effects in self-stimulation. J.Comp.Physiol. Psychol. **62**:96-101.

198. Gallistel, C. R. (1973) Self-stimulation: The neurophysiology of reward and motivation. In: Deutsch, J. A. (*Ed.*): The Physiological Basis of Memory. Academic Press, New York.

199. Garcia, J. and Kimeldorf, D. J. (1957) Temporal relationship within the conditioning of a saccharine aversion through radiation exposure. J.Comp. Physiol.Psychol. **50**:180-183.

200. Garcia, J. and Koelling, R. A. (1967) A comparison of aversions induced by X-rays, toxins and drugs in the rat. Radiation Res. **Suppl.7**:439-450.

201. Garris, P. A., Kilpatrick, M., Bunin, M. A., Michael, D., Walker, Q. D., and Wightman, R. M. (1999) Dissociation of dopamine release in the nucleus accumbens from intracranial self-stimulation. Nature **368**:67-69.

202. Gauvin, D. V., Briscoe, R. J., Baird, T. J., Vallett, M., and Holloway, F. A. (1997) The paradoxical hedonic valence of acute ethanol withdrawal (hangover) states in rats: Place and taste conditioning. Alcohol **14**:261-268.

203. Gerber, G. J., Bozarth, M. A., Spindler, J. E., and Wise, R. A. (1985) Concurrent heroin self-administration and intracranial self-stimulation in rats. Pharmacol.Biochem.Behav. **23**:837-842.

204. Ghatan, P. H., Ingvar, M., Eriksson, L., Stone-Elander, S., Serrander, M., Ekberg, K., and Wahren, J. (1998) Cerebral effects of nicotine during cognition in smokers and non-smokers. Psychopharmacology **136**:179-189.

205. Gibbons, F. X., Gerrard, M., Blanton, H., and Russell, D. W. (1998) Reasoned action and social reaction: Willingness and intention as independent predictors of health risk. J.Person.Soc.Psychol. **74**:1164-1180.

206. Gibson, W. E., Reid, L. D., Sakai, M., and Porter, P. B. (1965) Intracranial reinforcement compared with sugar water reinforcement. Science **148**:1357- 1359.

207. Gillholm, R., Erdeus, J., and Gaerling, T. (2000) The effect of choice on intention-behavior consistency. Scand.J.Psychol. **41**:1-8.

208. Gillin, J. C., Lardon, M., Ruiz, C., Golshan, S., and Salin-Pascual, R. (1994) Dose-dependent effects of transdermal nicotine on early morning awakening and rapid eye movement sleep time in nonsmoking normal volunteers. J.Clin. Psychopharmacol. **14**:264-267.

209. Giorgi, O., Corda, M. G., Carboni, G., Frau, V., Valentini, V., and DiChiara, G. (1997) Effects of cocaine and morphine in rats from 2 psychogenetically selected lines - a behavioral and brain dialysis study. Behav.Genet. **27**:537-546.

210. Glasgow, R. E., Cummings, K. M., and Hyland, A. (1997) Relationship of worksite smoking policy to changes in employee tobacco use: Findings from COMMIT. Community Intervention Trial for Smoking Cessation. Tobacco Control **6 Suppl. 2**:S44-S48.

211. Glick, S. D., Maisonneuve, I. M., Visker, K. E., Fritz, K. A., Bandarage, U. K., and Kuehne, M. E. (1998) 18-Methoxycoronardine attenuates nicotine-induced dopamine release and nicotine preferences in rats. Psychopharmacology **139**:274-280.

212. Glick, S. D., Visker, K. E., and Maisonneuve, I. M. (1996) An oral self-administration model of nicotine preference in rats: Effects of mecamylamine. Psychopharmacology **128**:426-431.

213. Glick, S. D., Weaver, L. M., and Meibach, R. C. (1982) Asymmetrical effects of morphine and naloxone on reward mechanisms. Psychopharmacology **78**:219-224.

214. Goldberg, S. R. and Henningfield, J. E. (1983) Fixed-ratio responding maintained by intravenous nicotine injections in humans and squirrel monkeys. Pharmacologist **25**:219.

215. Goldberg, S. R. and Henningfield, J. E. (1983) Intravenous nicotine self-administration in humans and squirrel monkeys. Neurosci.Lett. **14(Suppl.)**:S140.

216. Goldberg, S. R. and Henningfield, J. E. (1986) Nicotine as a reinforcer in humans and experimental animals. Paper presented at symposium on Progress in Understanding the Relationship Between the Pharmacological Effects of Nicotine and Human Tobacco Dependence, held at annual meeting of American Society for Pharmacology and Experimental Therapeutics. Baltimore, MD. (C.f. US Department of Health and Human Services, 1988),

217. Goldberg, S. R. and Henningfield, J. E. (1988) Reinforcing effects of nicotine in humans and experimental animals responding under intermittent schedules of i.v. drug injection. Pharmacol.Biochem.Behav. **30**:227-234.

218. Goldberg, S. R., Risner, M. E., Stolerman, I. P., Reavill, C., and Garcha, H. S. (1989) Nicotine and some related compounds: Effects on schedule-controlled behaviour and discriminative properties in rats. Psychopharmacology **97**:295-302.

219. Goldberg, S. R. and Spealman, R. D. (1982) Maintenance and suppression of behavior by intravenous nicotine injections in squirrel monkeys. Fed.Proc. **41**: 216-220.

220. Goldberg, S. R., Spealman, R. D., and Goldberg, D. M. (10-30-1981) Persistent behavior at high rates maintained by intravenous self-administration of nicotine. Science **214**:573-575.

221. Goldfarb, T., Gritz, E. R., Jarvik, M. E., and Stolerman, I. P. (1976) Reactions to cigarettes as a function of nicotine and "tar". Clin.Pharmacol.Ther. **19**:768-772.

222. Gollwitzer, P. M. and Bargh, J. E. (1996) The Psychology of Action: Linking Cognition and Motivation to Behavior. The Guilford Press, New York.

223. Gollwitzer, P. M. and Brandstaetter, V. (1997) Implementation intentions and effective goal pursuit. J.Person.Soc.Psychol. **73**:186-199.

224. Goode, E. (1989) Drugs in American Society, 3. Knopf, New York.

225. Goodman, W. K., Price, L. H., Rasmussen, S. A., Mazure, C., Fleischmann, R. L., Hill, C. L., Heninger, G. R., and Charney, D. S. (1989) The Yale-Brown Obsessive Compulsive Scale: I. Development, use, and reliability. Arch.Gen. Psychiatry **6**:1006-1011.

226. Gordon, F. J. and Johnson, A. K. (1981) Electrical stimulation of the septal area in the rat: Prolonged suppression of water intake and correlation with self- stimulation. Brain Res. **206**:421-430.

227. Gorelick, D. A., Rose, J., and Jarvik, M. E. (1989) Effect of naloxone on cigarette smoking. J.Subst.Abuse **1**:153-159.

228. Gori, G. B. and Lynch, C. J. (1985) Analytical cigarette yields as predictors of smoke bioavailability. Regul.Toxicol.Pharmacol. **5**:314-326.

229. Grant, S. G. N., Pavia, D., and Clarke, S. W. (1982) Relationship of lung smoke exposure to cigarette nicotine. Am.Rev.Respir.Dis. **125**:153.

230. Gray, J. A., Young, A. M., and Joseph, M. H. (1997) Dopamine's role [letter]. Science **278**:1548-1549.

231. Green, J. T., Thomas, G. A. O., Rhodes, J., Evans, B. K., Russell, M. A., Feyerabend, C., Fuller, G. S., Newcombe, R. G., and Sandborn, W. J. (1997) Pharmacokinetics of nicotine carbomer enemas: A new treatment modality for ulcerative colitis. Clin.Pharmacol.Ther. **61**:340-348.

232. Greenland, S., Satterfield, M. H., and Lanes, S. F. (1998) A meta-analysis to assess the incidence of adverse effects associated with the transdermal nicotine patch. Drug Saf. **18**:297-308.

233. Greiff, L., Wollmer, P., Andersson, M., Pipkom, U., and Persson, C. G. A. (1993) Effects of nicotine on the human nasal mucosa. Thorax **48**:651-655.

234. Griffiths, R. R., Brady, J. V., and Bradford, L. D. (1979) Predicting the abuse liability of drugs with animal drug self-administration procedures: Psychomotor stimulants and hallucinogens. In: Thompson, T. and Dews, P. B. (*Eds.*): Advances in Behavioral Pharmacology, Volume 2. Academic Press, New York.

235. Grigson, P. S. (1997) Conditioned taste aversions and drugs of abuse: A reinterpretation. Behav.Neurosci. **111**:129-136.

236. Grodstein, F., Levine, R., Troy, L., Spencer, T., Colditz, G. A., and Stampfer, M. J. (1996) Three-year follow-up of participants in a commercial weight loss program. Arch.Intern.Med. **156**:1302-1306.

237. Gross, J., Johnson, J., Sigler, L., and Stitzer, M. L. (1995) Dose effects of nicotine gum. Addict.Behav. **20**:371-381.

238. Gross, J., Lee, J., and Stitzer, M. L. (1997) Nicotine-containing versus de-nicotinized cigarettes: Effects on craving and withdrawal. Pharmacol. Biochem.Behav. **57**:159-165.

239. Gross, J. and Stitzer, M. L. (1989) Nicotine replacement: Ten-week effects on tobacco withdrawal symptoms. Psychopharmacology **98**:334-341.

240. Gunnar, M. G., Fisch, R. O., and Malone, S. (1984) The effects of a pacifying stimulus on behavioral and adrenocortical responses to circumcision in the newborn. J.Am.Acad.Child Psychiat. **23**:34-38.

241. Guslandi, M. and Tittobello, A. (1996) Pilot trial of nicotine patches as an alternative to corticosteroids in ulcerative colitis. J.Gastroenterol. **31**:627-629.

242. Gust, S. W. and Pickens, R. W. (1982) Does cigarette nicotine yield affect puff volume? Clin.Pharmacol.Ther. **32**:418-422.

243. Gybels, J. (1999) The placebo effect: Classes of explanation (in Dutch). Verh.K. Acad.Geneeskd.Belg. **61**:1-17.

244. Haertzen, C. A. (1966) Development of scales based on patterns of drug effects using the Addiction Research Center Inventory (ARCI). Psychol.Rep. **18**:163-194.

245. Hajek, P., Jackson, P., and Belcher, M. (1988) Long-term use of nicotine chewing gum. Occurrence, determinants, and effect of weight gain. JAMA **260**:1593-1596.

246. Hajek, P., West, R., Foulds, J., Nilsson, F., Burrows, S., and Meadow, A. (1999) Randomized comparative trail of nicotine polacrilex, a transdermal patch, nasal spray, and an inhaler. Arch.Intern.Med. **159**:2033-2038.

247. Hajek, P., West, R., and Wilson, J. (1995) Regular smokers, lifetime very light smokers, and reduced smokers: Comparison of psychosocial and smoking characteristics in women. Hlth.Psychol. **14**:195-201.

248. Hakan, T. (1988) Nictone-induced locomotor activity in rats. Pharmacol. Biochem. Behav. **29**:661-663.

249. Haley, N. J., Sepkovic, W., Hoffman, D., and Wynder, E. L. (1985) Cigarette smoking as a risk for cardiovascular disease. Part VI. Compensation with nicotine availability as a single variable. Clin.Pharmacol.Ther. **38**:164-170.

250. Hall, S. M., Munoz, R. F., Reus, V. I., Sees, K. L., Duncan, C., Humfleet, G. L., and Hartz, D. T. (1996) Mood management and nicotine gum in smoking treatment: A therapeutic contact and placebo-controlled study. J.Counsel.Clin. Psychol. **64**:1003-1009.

251. Hamid, A., Curtis, R., McCoy, K., McGuire, J., Conde, A., Bushell, W., Lindenmayer, R., Brimberg, K., Maia, S., Abdur-Rashid, S., and Settembrino, J. (1997) The heroin epidemic in New York City: Current status and prognosis. J.Psychoactive Drugs **29**:375-391.

252. Hand, T. H. and Franklin, K. B. (1986) Associative factors in the effects of morphine on self-stimulation. Psychopharmacology **88**:472-479.

253. Hanson, H. M., Ivester, C. A., and Morton, B. R. (1979) Nicotine self-administration in rats. NIDA Res.Monogr 70-90.

254. Harrington, G. M. (1979) Strain differences in light-contingent barpress behavior of the rat. Bulletin of the Psychonomic Society **13**:155-156.

255. Hasenfratz, M., Baldinger, B., and Battig, K. (1993) Nicotine or tar titration in cigarette smoking behavior? Psychopharmacology **112**:253-258.

256. Hasenfratz, M., Pfiffner, D., Pellaud, K., and Battig, K. (1989) Postlunch smoking for pleasure seeking or arousal maintenance? Pharmacol.Biochem. Behav. **34**:631-639.

257. Hatsukami, D., Huber, M., Callies, A., and Skoog, K. (1993) Physical dependence on nicotine gum: Effect of duration of use. Psychopharmacology **111**:449-456.

258. Hatsukami, D. K., Skoog, K., Huber, M., and Hughes, J. (1991) Signs and symptoms from nicotine gum abstinence. Psychopharmacology **104**:496-504.

259. Heishman, S. J., Snyder, B. J., and Henningfield, J. E. (1993) Performance, subjective, and physiological effects of nicotine in non-smokers. Drug Alc. Depend. **34**:11-18.

260. Helton, D. R., Modlin, D. L., Tizzano, J. P., and Rasmussen, K. (1993) Nicotine withdrawal: A behavioral assessment using schedule controlled responding, locomotor activity, and sensorimotor reactivity. Psychopharmacology **113**:205-210.

261. Helton, D. R., Tizzano, J. P., Monn, J. A., Schoepp, D. D., and Kallman, M. J. (1997) LY354740: A metabotropic glutamate receptor agonist which ameliorates symptoms of nicotine withdrawal in rats. Neuropharmacol. **36**:1511-1516.

262. Hendry, J. S. and Rosecrans, J. A. (1982) The development of pharmacological tolerance to the effects of schedule-controlled responding in mice. Psycho-pharmacology **77**:339-343.

263. Henningfield, J. E., Benowitz, N. L., Slade, J., Houston, T. P., Davis, R. M., and Deitchman, S. D. (1998) Reducing the addictiveness of cigarettes. Presentation by the AMA Council on Scientific Affairs to the AMA House of Delegates at its 147th annual meeting.

264. Henningfield, J. E. and Goldberg, S. R. (1983) Control of behavior by intravenous nicotine injections in human subjects. Pharmacol.Biochem.Behav. **19**:1021-1026.

265. Henningfield, J. E. and Keenan, R. M. (1993) Nicotine delivery kinetics and abuse liability. J.Cons.Clin.Psychol. **61**:743-750.

266. Henningfield, J. E., Miyasato, K., and Jasinski, D. R. (1983) Cigarette smokers self-administer intravenous nicotine . Pharmacol.Biochem.Behav. **19**:887-890.

267. Henningfield, J. E., Miyasato, K., and Jasinski, D. R. (1985) Abuse liability and pharmacodynamic characteristics of intravenous and inhaled nicotine. J.Pharmacol.exp.Ther. **234**:1-12.

268. Henningfield, J. E. and Nemeth-Coslett, G. (1988) Nicotine dependence: Interface between tobacco and tobacco-related disease. Chest **93**:37S-55S.

269. Henningfield, J. E., Schuh, L. M., and Heishman, S. J. (1995) Pharmacological determinants of cigarette smoking. In: Clark, P. B. S., Quik, M., and Adlkofer, F. X. Thurau K. (*Eds.*): Effects of Nicotine on Biological Systems II. International Symposium on Nicotine Advances in Pharmacological Sciences. Birkhauser Verlag, Basel.

270. Hepper, P. G., Shahidullah, S., and White, R. (1991) Handedness in the human fetus. Neuropsychologia **29**:1107-1111.

271. Herberg, L. J. (1963) Seminal ejaculation following positively reinforcing electrical stimulation of the rat hypothalamus. J.Comp.Physiol.Psychol. **56**: 679-685.

272. Herberg, L. J., Montgomery, A. M. J., and Rose, I. C. (1993) Tolerance and sensitization to stimulant and depressant effects of nicotine in intra-cranial self-stimulation in the rat. Behav.Pharmacol. **4**:419-427.

273. Herning, R. I., Jones, R. T., Benowitz, N., and Mines, A. H. (1981) Puff volume increases when low-nicotine cigarettes are smoked. Br.Med.J. **283**:187-189.

274. Herning, R. I., Jones, R. T., and Fischman, P. (1985) The titration hypothesis revisited: Nicotine gum reduces smoking intensity. In: Grabowski, J. and Hall, S. M. (*Eds.*): Pharmacological Adjuncts in Smoking Cessation, NIDA Research Monograph Vol. 53. US Department of Health and Human Services,

275. Herzog, D. B., Dorer, D. J., Keel, P. K., Selwyn, S. E., Ekeblad, E. R., Flores, A. T., Greenwood, D. N., Burwell, R. A., and Keller, M. B. (1999) Recovery and relapse in anorexia and bulimia nervosa: A 7.5-year follow-up study. J.Acad. Child Adolesc.Psychiat. **38**:829-837.

276. Higgins, G. A., Wang, Y., Corrigall, W. A., and Sellers, E. M. (1994) Influence of the 5-HT3 receptor antagonists and the indirect 5-HT agonist, dexfenfluramine, on heroin self-administration in rats. Psychopharmacology **114**:611-619.

277. Hildebrand, B. E., Nomikos, G. G., Bondjers, C., Nisell, M., and Svensson, T. H. (1997) Behavioral manifestations of the nicotine abstinence syndrome in the rat: Peripheral versus central mechanisms. Psychopharmacology **129**:348-356.

278. Hill, P., Haley, N. J., and Wynder, E. L. (1983) Cigarette smoking: Carboxy-hemoglobin, plasma nicotine, cotinine and thiocyanate vs. self-reported smoking data and cardiovascular disease. J.Chron.Dis. **36**:439-449.

279. Hill, P. and Marquardt, H. (1980) Plasma and urine changes after smoking different brands of cigarettes. Clin.Pharmacol.Ther. **27**:652-658.

280. Hjalmarson, A., Franzon, M., and Westin, A. (1995) Effect of nicotine nasal spray on smoking cessation: A randomized, placebo controlled, double-blind study. Arch.Intern.Med. **154**:2567-2572.

281. Hoebel, B. G. and Teitelbaum, P. (1962) Hypothalamic control of feeding and self-stimulation. Science **135**:375-377.

282. Hofer, I., Nil, R., and Battig, K. (1991) Nicotine yield as determinent of smoke exposure indicators and puffing behavior. Pharmacol.Biochem.Behav. **40**:139- 149.

283. Hoffmann, D. and Hoffmann, I. (1997) The changing cigarette, 1950-1995. J.Toxicol.Environ.Hlth. **50**:307-364.

284. Holden, J. H., Darga, L. L., Olson, S. M., Stettner, D. D., Ardito, E. A., and Lucas, C. P. (1992) Long-term follow-up of patients attending a combination very-low calorie diet and behaviour therapy weight loss programme. Int.J.Obes. Relat.Metab. Disord. **16**:605-613.

285. Hollander, E. (1998) Treatment of obsessive-compulsive spectrum disorders with SSRIs . Br.J.Psychiat. **173 (Suppl.35)**:7-12.

286. Horan, B., Smith, M., Gardner, E. L., Lepore, M., and Ashby, C. R. (1997) (-)-Nicotine produces conditioned place preference in Lewis, but not Fischer 344 rats. Synapse **26**:93-94.

287. Horne, D. J. and Wilkinson, J. (1980) Habit reversal for fingernail biting. Behav. Res.Ther. **18**:287-291.

288. Hubbard, J. E. and Gohd, R. S. (1975) Tolerance development to the arousal effects of nicotine. Pharmacol.Biochem.Behav. **3**:471-476.

289. Hubner, C. B. and Kornetsky, C. (1992) Heroin, 6-acetylmorphine and morphine effects on threshold for rewarding and aversive brain stimulation. J.Pharmacol. exp.Ther. **260**:562-567.

290. Hudzinski, L. G. and Sirois, P. A. (1994) Changes in smoking-behavior and body-weight after implementation of a no-smoking policy in the workplace. Southern Med.J. **87**:322-327.

291. Hughes, J. R. (1987) Craving as a dependent variable. Br.J.Addict. **82**:483-484.

292. Hughes, J. R. (1989) Dependence potential and abuse liability of nicotine replacement therapies. Biomed.Pharmacother. **43**:11-17.

293. Hughes, J. R. (1992) Tobacco withdrawal in self-quitters. J.Cons.Clin.Psychol. **60**:689-697.

294. Hughes, J. R., Higgins, S. T., and Bickel, W. K. (1994) Nicotine withdrawal versus other drug withdrawal syndromes: Similarities and dissimilarities. Addiction **89**:1461-1470.

295. Hughes, J. R., Pickens, R. W., Spring, W., and Keenan, R. M. (1985) Instructions control whether nicotine will serve as a reinforcer. J.Pharmacol. exp.Ther. **235**:106-112.

296. Hughes, J. R., Strickler, G., King, D., Higgins, S. T., Fenwick, J. F., Gulliver, S. B., and Mireault, G. (1989) Smoking history, instructions and the effects of nicotine: Two pilot studies. Pharmacol.Biochem.Behav. **34**:149-155.

297. Hummel, T., Livermore, A., Hummel, C., and Kobal, G. (1992) Chemosensory event-related potentials in man: Relation to the olfactory and painful sensations elicited by nicotine. EEG.Clin.Neurophysiol. **84**:192-195.

298. Hurt, R. D., Offord, K. P., Lauger, G. G., Marusic, Z., Fagerstrom, K. O., Enright, P. L., and Scanlon, P. D. (1995) Cessation of long-term nicotine gum use - prospective, randomized trial. Addiction **90**:407-413.

299. Huston-Lyons, D. and Kornetsky, C. (1992) Effects of nicotine on the threshold for rewarding brain stimulation in rats. Pharmacol.Biochem.Behav. **41**:755-759.

300. Huston-Lyons, D., Sarkar, M., and Kornetsky, C. (1993) Nicotine and brain-stimulation reward: Interactions with morphine, amphetamine and pimozide. Pharmacol.Biochem.Behav. **46**:453-457.

301. Hutchinson, R. R. and Emley, G. S. (1988) Aversive stimulation produces nicotine ingestion in squirrel monkeys. Psychol.Rec. **35**:491-502.

302. Imperato, A., Angelucci, L., Casolini, P., Zocchi, A., and Puglisi-Allegra, S. (1992) Repeated stressful experiences differently affect limbic dopamine release during and following stress. Brain Res. **577**:194-199.

303. Imperato, A., Mulus, A., and DiChiara, G. (1986) Nicotine preferentially stimulates dopamine release in the limbic system of freely moving rats. Eur.J.Pharmacol. **132**:337-338.

304. Imperato, A., Puglisi-Allegra, S., Casolini, P., and Angelucci, L. (1991) Changes in brain dopamine and acetycholine release during and following stress are independent of the pituitary-adrenocortical axis. Brain Res. **538**:111-117.

305. Isbell, H. (1958) Clinical research on addiction in the United States. In: Livingston, R. B. (*Eds.*): Narcotic Drug Addiction Problems. Public Health Service, Bethesda, MD.

306. Ivanova, S. and Greenshaw, A. J. (1997) Nicotine-induced decreases in VTA electrical self-stimulation thresholds: Blockade by haloperidol and mecamylamine but not scopolamine or odansetron. Psychopharmacology **134**: 187-192.

307. Iwamoto, K. and Klaassen, C. D. (1977) First-pass effect of morphine in rat. J.Pharmacol.exp.Ther. **200**:236-244.

308. Izenwasser, S. E. and Kornetsky, C. (1987) Pharmacological effects of morphine on brain-stimulation reward [letter]. Psychopharmacology **93**:136-137.

309. Jackler, F., Steiner, S. S., Bodnar, R. J., Ackermann, R. F., Nelson, W. T., and Ellman, S. J. (1979) Morphine and intracranial self-stimulation in the hypothalamus and dorsal brainstem: Differential effects of dose, time and site. Int.J.Neurosci. **9**:21-35.

310. Jaffe, A. J. and Glaros, A. G. (1986) Taste dimensions in cigarette discrimination: A multidimensional scaling approach. Addict.Behav. **11**:407- 413.

311. Jaffe, J. (1990) Drug addiction and drug abuse. In: Goodman Gilman, A., Rall, T. W., Nies, A. S., and Taylor, P. (*Eds.*): Goodman and Gilman's The Pharmacological Basis of Therapeutics. Pergamon Press, New York.

312. Jaffe, J. H. and Martin, W. R. (1990) Opioid analgetics and antagonists. In: Goodman Gilman, A., Rall, T. W., Nies, A. S., and Taylor, P. (*Eds.*): Goodman and Gilman's The Pharmacological Basis of Therapeutics. Pergamon Press, New York.

313. James, W. (1890) The Principles of Psychology. Holt, New York.

314. Jansco, N., Jansco-Gabor, A., and Takats, I. (1961) Pain and inflammation induced by nicotine, acetylcholine and structurally related compounds and their prevention by desensitizing agents. Acta Physiol. **19**:113-132.

315. Jarvik, M., Killen, J. D., Varady, A., and Fortmann, S. P. (1993) The favorite cigarette of the day. J.Behav.Med. **16**:413-422.

316. Jarvik, M. E. (1991) Beneficial effects of nicotine. Br.J.Addict. **86**:571-575.

317. Jarvik, M. E. and Assil, K. M. (1988) Mecamylamine blocks the burning sensation of nicotine on the tongue. Chem.Senses **13**:213-217.

318. Jarvik, M. E., Saniga, S. S., Herskovic, J. E., Weiner, H., and Oisboid, D. (1989) Potentiation of cigarette craving and satisfaction by two types of meal. Addict.Behav. **14**:35-41.

319. Jeffery, R. W., Kelder, S. H., Forster, J. L., French, S. A., Lando, H. A., and Baxter, J. E. (1994) Restrictive smoking policies in the workplace - effects on smoking prevalence and cigarette consumption. Prevent.Med. **23**:78-82.

320. Jenkins, O. F., Atrens, D. M., and Jackson, D. M. (1983) Self-stimulation of the nucleus accumbens and some comparisons with hypothalamic self-stimulation. Pharmacol.Biochem.Behav. **18**:585-591.

321. Jenks, R. J. (1994) Attitudes and perceptions toward smoking: Smokers' views of themselves and other smokers. J.Soc.Psychol. **134**:355-361.

322. Jerome, A. and Sandberg, P. R. (1987) The effects of nicotine on locomotor behavior in non-tolerant rats: A multivariate assesment. Psychopharmacology **93**:397-400.

323. Johnston, C. C. (1989) Pain assessment and management in infants. Pediatrician **16**:23.

324. Jones, G. M. M., Sahakian, B. J., Levy, R., Warburton, D. M., and Gray, J. A. (1992) Effects of acute subcutaneous nicotine on attention, information processing and short-term memory in Alzheimer's disease. Psychopharmacology **108**:485-494.

325. Jones, R. T., Farrell, T. R, IIIrd, and Herning, R. I. (1978) Tobacco smoking and nicotine tolerance. In: Krasnegor, N. A. (*Ed.*): Self-Administration of Abused Substances: Methods for Study, NIDA Research Monograph 20. U.S. Department of Health, Education and Welfare, Public Health Service, Alcohol, Drug Abuse, and Mental Health Administration, National Institute on Drug Abuse,

326. Jorenby, D. E., Hatsukami, D. K., Smith, S. S., Fiore, M. C., Allen, S., Jensen, J., and Baker, T. B. (1996) Characterization of tobacco withdrawal symptoms: Transdermal nicotine reduces hunger and weight gain. Psychopharmacology **128**:130-138.

327. Jorenby, D. E., Smith, S. S., Fiore, M. C., Hurt, R. D., Offord, K. P., Croghan, I. T., Hays, J. T., Lewis, S. F., and Baker, T. B. (1995) Varying nicotine patch dose and type of smoking cessation counseling. JAMA **274**:1347-1352.

328. Jorenby, D. E., Steinpreis, R. E., Sherman, J. E., and Baker, T. B. (1990) Aversion instead of preference learning indicated by nicotine place conditioning in rats. Psychopharmacology **101**:533-538.

329. Joseph, M. H., Young, A. M. J., and Gray, J. A. (1996) Are neurochemistry and reinforcement enough – can the abuse potential of drugs be explained by common actions on a dopamine reward system in the brain? Human Psychopharmacol. **11**:55-63.

330. Kamei, C. (1994) Changes in self-stimulation response during chronic morphine treatment and after withdrawal of morphine in rats. Jpn.J.Pharmacol. **66**:163-165.

331. Kanarek, R. B. and Collier, G. H. (1983) Self-starvation: A problem of overriding the satiety signal? Physiol.Behav. **30**:307-311.

332. Kandel, D. B. (1975) Stages in adolescent involvement in drug use. Science **190**:912-914.

333. Karras, A. and Kane, K. (1980) Naloxone reduces cigarette smoking. Life Sci. **27**:1541-1545.

334. Katz, R. C. and Singh, N. N. (1986) Reflections on the ex-smoker: Some findings on successful quitters. J.Behav.Med. **9**:191-202.

335. Katz, R. J. and Roth, K. (1979) Tail pinch induced stress-arousal facilitates brain stimulation reward. Physiol.Behav. **22**:193-194.

336. Katz, R. J., Roth, K. A., and Schmaltz, K. (1980) Tail-pinch facilitation of self-stimulation in the rat - dependence upon dopamine and independence of opiates. Pharmacol.Biochem.Behav. **12**:389-391.

337. Kavaliers, M., Colwell, D. D., Choleris, E., and Ossenkopp, K. P. (1999) Learning to cope with biting flies: Rapid NMDA-mediated acquisition of conditioned analgesia. Behav.Neurosci. **113**:126-135.

338. Keel, P. K. and Mitchell, J. E. (1997) Outcome in bulimia nervosa. Am.J.Psychiat. **154**:313-321.

339. Kendzierski, D. (1990) Decision making versus decision implementation: An action control approach to exercise adoption and adherence. J.Appl.Psychol. **20**:27-45.

340. Kendzierski, D. and Whitaker, D. J. (1997) The role of self-schema in linking intentions with behavior. Person.Soc.Psychol.Bull. **23**:139-147.

341. Kennedy, L. D. (1996) Nicotine therapy for ulcerative colitis. Ann. Pharmacother. **30**:1022-1023.

342. Kent, E. and Grossman, S. P. (1969) Evidence for a conflict interpretation of anomalous effects of rewarding brain stimulation. J.Comp.Physiol.Psychol. **69**: 381-390.

343. Killian, A. K., Bonese, K., and Schuster, C. R. (1978) The effects of naloxone on behavior maintained by cocaine and heroin injections in the rhesus monkey. Drug Alc.Depend. **3**:243-251.

344. Kitano, T. and Takemori, A. E. (1977) Enhanced affinity of opiate receptors for naloxone in striatal slices of morphine-dependent mice. Res.Commun.Chem. Pathol. Pharmacol. **18**:341-351.

345. Knapp, C. M. and Kornetsky, C. (1996) Low-dose apomorphine attenuates morphine-induced enhancement of brain stimulation reward. Pharmacol. Biochem.Behav. **55**:87-91.

346. Knott, P. D. and Clayton, K. N. (1966) Durable secondary reinforcement using brain stimulation as the primary reinforcer. J.Comp.Physiol.Psychol. **61**:151- 153.

347. Knott, V., Bosman, M., Mahoney, C., Illivitsky, V., and Quirt, K. (1999) Transdermal nicotine: Single dose effects on mood, EEG, performance, and event-related potentials. Pharmacol.Biochem.Behav. **63**:253-261.

348. Kolonen, S., Tuomisto, J., Puustinen, P., and Airaksinen, M. M. (1991) Smoking behavior in low-yield cigarette smokers and switchers in the natural environment. Pharmacol.Biochem.Behav. **40**:177-180.

349. Kolonen, S., Tuomisto, J., Puustinen, P., and Airaksinen, M. M. (1992) Puffing behavior during the smoking of a single cigarette in a naturalistic environment. Pharmacol.Biochem.Behav. **41**:701-706.

350. Koob, G. F., Petit, H. O., Ettenberg, A., and Bloom, F. E. (1984) Effects of opiate antagonists and their quarternary derivatives on heroin self-administration in the rat. J.Pharmacol.exp.Ther. **229**:481-486.

351. Korhonen, T., Su, S., Korhonen, H. J., Uutela, A., and Puska, P. (1997) Evaluation of a national Quit and Win contest: Determinants for successful quitting. Prevent. Med. **26**:556-564.

352. Kornblith, C. and Olds, J. (1968) T-maze learning with one trial per day using brain stimulation reinforcement. J.Comp.Physiol.Psychol. **66**:488-492.

353. Kornetsky, C., Esposito, R. U., McLean, S., and Jacobson, J. O. (1979) Intracranial self-stimulation thresholds: A model for the hedonic effects of drugs of abuse. Arch.Gen.Psychiatry **36**:289-292.

354. Kornitzer, M., Boutsen, M., Dramaix, M., Thijs, J., and Gustavsson, G. (1995) Combined use of nicotine patch and gum in smoking cessation: A placebo-controlled clinical trial. Prevent.Med. **24**:41-47.

355. Kozlowski, L. T., Herman, C. P., and Frecker, R. C. (1980) What researchers make of what cigarette smokers say: Filtering smokers' hot air. The Lancet 699-700.

356. Kozlowski, L. T. and Wilkinson, D. A. (1987) Comments on Kozlowski and Wilkinson's "Use and misuse of the concept of craving by alcohol, tobacco, and drug researchers": A reply from the authors. Br.J.Addict. **82**:489-492.

357. Kramer, F. M., Jeffery, R. W., Forster, J. L., and Snell, M. K. (1989) Long-term follow-up of behavioral treatment of obesity: Patterns of regain among men and women. Int.J.Obes. **13**:123-136.

358. Kreek, M. J. (1997) Opiate and cocaine addictions: Challenge for pharmaco-therapies. Pharmacol.Biochem.Behav. **57**:551-569.

359. Kumar, R., Cooke, E. C., Lader, M. H., and Russell, M. A. H. (1977) Is nicotine important in tobacco smoking? Clin.Pharmacol.Ther. **21**:520-529.

360. Kumari, V., Cotter, P. A., Checkley, S. A., and Gray, J. A. (1997) Effect of acute subcutaneous nicotine on prepulse inhibition of the acoustic startle reflex in healthy male non-smokers. Psychopharmacology **132**:389-395.

361. Kuschinsky, G. and Hotovy, R. (1943) Ueber die zentral erregende Wirkung des Nicotins. Klin.Wochenschr. **22**:649-650.

362. Lacey, J. H., Coker, S., and Birtchnell, S. A. (1986) Bulimia: Factors associated with its etiology and maintenance. Int.J.Eating Disord. **5**:475-487.

363. Lakatos, I. (1970) Falsification and the methodology of scientific research programs. In: Lakatos, I. and Musgrave, A. (*Eds.*): Criticism and the Growth of Knowledge. Cambridge University Press, Cambridge.

364. Lakatos, I. (1977) Philosophical Papers, Vol. 1. Cambridge University Press, Cambridge.

365. Lakatos, I and Musgrave, A. (1970) Criticism and the Growth of Knowledge. Cambridge University Press, Cambridge.

366. Lang, W. J., Latiff, A. A., Mcqueen, A., and Singer, G. (1977) Self administration of nicotine with and without a food delivery schedule. Pharmacol. Biochem.Behav. 7:65-70.

367. LaPiere, R. (1934) Attitudes versus actions. Social Forces 13:230-237.

368. Lau, C. E., Spear, D. J., and Falk, J. L. (1994) Acute and chronic nicotine effects on multiple-schedule behavior: Oral and SC routes. Pharmacol.Biochem.Behav. 48:209-215.

369. Le Houezec, J. (1998) Nicotine: Abused substance and therapeutic agent. J.Psychiatry Neurosci. 23:95-108.

370. Le Houezec, J., Halliday, R., Benowitz, N. L., Callaway, E., Naylor, H., and Herzig, K. (1994) A low dose of subcutaneous nicotine improves information processing in non-smokers. Psychopharmacology 114:628-634.

371. Le Houezec, J., Jacob, P., and Benowitz, N. L. (1993) A clinical pharmacological study of subcutaneous nicotine. Eur.J.Clin.Pharmacol. 44:225-230.

372. LeBlanc, A. E. and Cappell, H. (1974) Attenuation of punishing effects of morphine and amphetaine by chronic prior treatment. J.Comp.Physiol.Psychol. 87:691-698.

373. Leischow, S. J., Valente, S. N., Hill, A. L., Otte, P. S., Aickin, M., Holden, T., Kligman, E., and Cook, G. (1997) Effects of nicotine dose and administration method on withdrawal symptoms and side effects during short-term smoking abstinence. Exp.Clin.Psychopharmacol. 5:54-64.

374. Lennox, A. S. and Taylor, R. J. (1994) Factors associated with outcome in unaided smoking cessation, and a comparison of those who have never tried to stop with those who have. Br.J.Gen.Practice. 44:245-250.

375. Lerner, J., Franklin, M. E., Meadows, E. A., Hembree, E., and Foa, E. B. (1998) Effectiveness of a cognitive behavioral treatment program for trichotillomania: An uncontrolled evaluation. Behav.Ther. 29:157-171.

376. Lett, B. T. and Grant, V. L. (1996) Wheel running induces conditioned taste aversion in rats trained while hungry and thirsty. Physiol.Behav. 59:699-702.

377. Lett, B. T., Grant, V. L., Neville, L. L., Davis, M. J., and Koh, M. T. (1997) Chlordiazepoxide counteracts activity-induced suppression of eating in rats. Exp.Clin.Psychopharmacol. 5:24-27.

378. Levin, E. D. (1992) Nicotinic systems and cognitive function. Psychopharmacology 108:417-431.

379. Levin, E. D., Conners, C. K., Silva, D., Hinton, S. C., Meck, W. H., March, J., and Rose, J. E. (1998) Transdermal nicotine effects on attention. Psycho- pharmacology **140**:135-141.

380. Levin, E. D., Morgan, M. M., Galvez, C., and Ellison, G. D. (1987) Chronic nicotine and withdrawal effects on body weight and food and water consumption in female rats. Physiol.Behav. **39**:441-444.

381. Levin, E. D., Rose, J. E., and Behm, F. (1990) Development of a citric aerosal as a smoking cessation aid. Drug Alc.Depend. **25**:279.

382. Levin, E. D. and Simon, B. R. (1998) Nicotinic acetylcholine involvement in cognitive function in animals. Psychopharmacology **138**:217-230.

383. Levin, E. D., Westman, E. C., Stein, R. M., Carnahan, E., Sanchez, M., Herman, S., Behm, F. M., and Rose, J. E. (1994) Nicotine skin patch treatment increases abstinence, decreases withdrawal symptoms, and attenuates rewarding effects of smoking. J.Clin.Psychopharmacol. **14**:41-49.

384. Levine, H. G. (1978) The discovery of addiction: Changing conceptions of habitual drunkenness in America. J.Studies Alcoholism **39**:143-174.

385. Liebman, J. M. (1985) Anxiety, anxiolytics and brain stimulation reinforcement. Neurosci.Biobehav.Rev. **9**:75-86.

386. Light, A. B. and Torrance, E. G. (1929) Opiate addiction VI: The effects of abrupt withdrawal followed by readministration of morphine in human addicts, with special reference to the composition of the blood, the circulation and the metabolism. Archives of Internal Medicine **44**:1-16.

387. Lorens, S. A. (1976) Comparison of the effects of morphine on hypothalamic and medial frontal cortex self-stimulation in the rat. Psychopharmacology **48**:217-224.

388. Lorens, S. A. and Mitchell, C. L. (1973) Influence of morphine on lateral hypothalamic self-stimulation in the rat. Psychopharmacologia **32**:271-277.

389. Louis, M. and Clarke, P. B. (1998) Effect of ventral tegmental 6-hydroxydopamine lesions on the locomotor stimulant action of nicotine in rats. Neuropharmacol. **37**:1503-1513.

390. Lynch, W. J. and Carroll, M. E. (1999) Regulation of intravenously self-administered nicotine in rats. Exp.Clin.Psychopharmacol. **7**:198-207.

391. Madden, C., Oei, T. P., and Singer, G. (1980) The effect of schedule removal on the maintenance of heroin self-injection. Pharmacol.Biochem.Behav. **12**:983- 986.

392. Malin, D. H., Lake, J. R., Carter, V. A., Cunningham, J. S., Herbert, K. M., Conrad, D. L., and Wilson, O. B. (1994) The nicotinic antagonist mecamylamine precipitates nicotine abstinence syndrome in the rat. Psychopharmacology **115**:180-184.

393. Malin, D. H., Lake, J. R., Carter, V. A., Cunningham, J. S., and Wilson, O. B. (1993) Naloxone precipitates nicotine abstinence syndrome in the rat. Psychopharmacology **112**:339-342.

394. Malin, D. H., Lake, J. R., Newlin-Maultsby, P., Roberts, L. K., Lanier, J. G., Carter, V. A., Cunningham, J. S., and Wilson, O. B. (1992) Rodent model of nicotine abstinence syndrome. Pharmacol.Biochem.Behav. **43**:779-784.

395. Malin, D. H., Lake, J. R., Payne, M. C., Short, P. E., Carter, V. A., Cunningham, J. S., and Wilson, O. B. (1996) Nicotine alleviation of nicotine abstinence syndrome is naloxone-reversible. Pharmacol.Biochem.Behav. **53**:81-85.

396. Malin, D. H., Lake, J. R., Schopen, C. K., Kirk, J. W., Sailer, E. E., Lawless, B. A., Upchurch, T. P., Shenoi, M., and Rajan, N. (1997) Nicotine abstinence syndrome precipitated by central but not peripheral hexamethonium. Pharmacol.Biochem.Behav. **58**:695-699.

397. Malin, D. H., Lake, J. R., Shenoi, M., Upchurch, T. P., Johnson, S. S., Schweinle, W. E., and Cadle, C. D. (1998) The nitric oxide synthesis inhibitor nitro-L-arginine (L-NNA) attenuates nicotine abstinence syndrome in the rat. Psychopharmacology **140**:371-377.

398. Malin, D. H., Lake, J. R., Short, P. E., Blossman, J. B., Lawless, B. A., Schopen, C. K., Sailer, E. E., Burgess, K., and Wilson, O. B. (1996) Nicotine abstinence syndrome precipitated by an analog of neuropeptide FF. Pharmacol.Biochem. Behav. **54**:581-585.

399. Manning, B. H., Mao, J., Frenk, H., Price, D. D., and Mayer, D. J. (1976) Continuous co-administration of dextromethorphan or MK-801 with morphine: attenuation of morphine dependence and naloxone-reversible attenuation of morphine tolerance. Pain **67**:79-88.

400. Margules, D. L. and Olds, J. (1962) Identical "feeding" and "rewarding" systems in the lateral hypothalamus of rats. Science **135**:374-375.

401. Marinelli, M., Aouizerate, B., Barrot, M., Lemoal, M., and Piazza, P. V. (1998) Dopamine-dependent responses to morphine depend on glucocorticoid receptors. Proc.Nat.Acad.Sci.USA **95**:7742-7747.

402. Marks, I. (1987) Fears, Phobias, and Rituals. Oxford University Press, Oxford, England.

403. Marks, I. (1990) Behavioural (non-chemical) addictions. Br.J.Addict. **85**: 1389-1394.

404. Marlatt, G. A., Baer, J. S., Donovan, D. M., and Klivahan, D. (1988) Addictive behaviors: Etiology and treatment. Ann.Rev.Psychol. **39**:223-252.

405. Maron, D. J. and Fortmann, S. P. (1987) Nicotine yield and measures of cigarette smoke exposure in a large population: Are lower-yield cigarettes safer? Am.J. Pub.Health **77**:546-549.

406. Martellotta, M. C., Kuzmin, A., Zvartau, E., Cossu, G., Gessa, G. L., and Fratta, W. (1995) Isradipine inhibits nicotine intravenous self-administration in drug-naive mice. Pharmacol.Biochem.Behav. **52**:271-274.

407. Martin, D. S. (1990) Physical dependence and attributions of addiction among cigarette smokers. Addict.Behav. **15**:69-72.

408. Martin, T. J., Dworkin, S. I., and Smith, J. E. (1995) Alkylation of mu opioid receptors by beta-funaltrexamine in vivo: Comparison of the effects on the in situ binding and heroin self-administration in rats. J.Pharmacol.exp.Ther. **272**:1135-1140.

409. Martin, T. J., Smith, J. E., and Dworkin, S. I. (1998) Training dose and session time as contextual determinants of heroin self-administration in rats. Pharmacol. Biochem.Behav. **60**:415-421.

410. Martin, T. J., Walker, L. E., Sizemore, G. M., Smith, J. E., and Dworkin, S. I. (1996) Within-session determination of dose-response curves for heroin self-administration in rats: Comparison with between-session determination and effects of naltrexone. Drug Alc.Depend. **41**:93-100.

411. McAughey, J., Black, A., Pritchard, J., and Knight, D. (1997) Measured tar deposition and compensation in smokers switching to lower yielding products. Ann.Occup.Hyg. **41**:719-723.

412. McCormick, R. A. and Taber, J. I. (1991) Follow-up of male pathological gamblers after treatment: The relationship of intellectual variables to relapse. J.Gambling Stud. **7**:99-108.

413. McGregor, I. S. and Atrens, D. M. (1990) Stressor-like effects of FG-7142 on medial prefrontal cortex self-stimulation. Brain Res. **516**:170-174.

414. McGregor, I. S., Balleine, B. W., and Atrens, D. M. (1989) Footshock stress facilitates self-stimulation of the medial prefrontal cortex but not the lateral hypothalamus in the rat. Brain Res. **490**:397-403.

415. McManus, F. and Waller, G. (1995) A functional analysis of binge-eating. Clin. Psychol.Rev. **15**:845-863.

416. McMorrow, M. and Foxx, R. M. (1983) Nicotine's role in smoking: An analysis of nicotine regulation. Psychol.Bull. **93**:302-327.

417. McNeill, A. D. (1991) The development of dependence on smoking in children. Br.J.Addict. **86**:589-592.

418. Melchiorri, P., Maritati, M., Negri, L., and Erspamer, V. (1992) Long-term sensitization to the activation of cerebral delta-opioid receptors by the dettorphin Tyr-D-Ala-Phe-Glu-Val-Val-Gly-NH2 in rats exposed to morphine. Proc.Nat. Acad. Sci.USA **89**:3696-3700.

419. Mendelson, J. (1967) Lateral hypothalamic stimulation in satiated rats: The rewarding effects of self-induced drinking. Science **157**:1077-1079.

420. Meyer, R. E. and Mirin, S. M. (1979) The Heroin Stimulus: Implications for a Study of Addiction. Plenum Press, New York.

421. Millar, W. J. and Bisch, L. M. (1989) Smoking in the working place 1986: Labour Force Survey estimates. Canadian Journal of Public Health **80**:261-265.

422. Miller, H. D. and Anderson, G. C. (1993) Nonnutritive sucking: Effects on crying and heart rate in intubated infants requiring assisted mechanical ventilation. Nursing Research **42**:305-307.

423. Miller, W. C. (1999) How effective are traditional dietary and exercise interventions for weight loss? Med.Sci.Sports and Exerc. **31**:1129-1134.

424. Milner, P. M. (1978) Test of two hypotheses about summation of rewarding brain stimulation. Canad.J.Psychol. **32** :95-105.

425. MMWR. (1999) Cigarette smoking among adults – United States, 1997. MMWR Morb.Mortal Wkly Rep. **48**:993-996.

426. Modell, J. G., Glaser, F. B., Cyr, L., and Mountz, J. M. (1992) Obsessive and compulsive characteristics of craving for alcohol in alcohol abuse and dependence. Alcoholism: Clinical and Experimental Research **16**:272-274.

427. Modell, J. G., Glaser, F. B., Mountz, J. M., Schmaltz, S., and Cyr, L. (1992) Obsessive and compulsive characteristics of craving of alcohol abuse and dependence: Quantification by a newly developed questionnaire. Alcoholism: Clinical and Experimental Research **16**:266-271.

428. Mogenson, G. J. and Stevenson, J. A. F. (1966) Drinking and self-stimulation with electrical stimulation of the lateral hypothalamus. Physiol.Behav. **1**:251-254.

429. Mokdad, A. H., Serdula, M. K., Dietz, W. H., Bowman, B. A., Marks, J. S., and Koplan, J. P. (1999) The spread of the obesity epidemic in the United States, 1991-1998. JAMA **282**:1519-1522.

430. Montague, P. R., Dayan, P., and Sejnowski, T. J. (1996) A framework for mesencephalic dopamine systems based on predictive Hebbian learning. J.Neurosci. **16**:1936-1947.

431. Montalto, N., Brackett, C. C., and Sobol, T. (1994) Use of transdermal nicotine systems in a possible suicide attempt. J.Am.Board Fam.Pract. **7** :417-420.

432. Morrison, C. F. (1967) Effects of nicotine on operant behaviour of rats. Int.J.Neuropharmac. **6**:229-240.

433. Morrison, C. F. and Stephenson, J. A. (1972) The occurrence of tolerance to a central depressant effect of nicotine. Br.J.Pharmac. **45**:151-156.

434. Moss, R. A. and Prue, D. M. (1982) Research on nicotine regulation. Behav.Ther. **13**:31-46.

435. Mucha, R. F. (1997) Preferences for tastes paired with a nicotine antagonist in rats chronically treated with nicotine. Pharmacol.Biochem.Behav. **56**:175-179.

436. Mucha, R. F., Van der Kooy, D., O'Shaughnessy, M., and Bucenieks, P. (1982) Drug reinforcement studied by the use of place conditioning in rat. Brain Res. **243**:91-105.

437. Mullis, K. (1998) Dancing Naked in the Mind Field. Pantheon Books, New York.

438. Museo, E. and Wise, R. A. (1990) Locomotion induced by ventral tegmental microinjections of a nicotine agonist. Pharmacol.Biochem.Behav. **35**:735-737.

439. Must, A., Spadano, J., Coakley, E. H., Field, A. E., Colditz, G., and Dietz, W. H. (1999) The disease burden associated with overweight and obesity. JAMA **282**: 1523-1529.

440. Myslobodsky, M. (1976) Petit Mal Epilepsy: A Search for the Precursors of Wave-Spike Activity. Academic Press, New York.

441. Nadal, R. and Samson, H. H. (1999) Operant ethanol self-administration after nicotine treatment and withdrawal. Alcohol **17**:139-147.

442. Nader, K., Bechara, A., and Van der Kooy, D. (1996) Lesions of the lateral prabrachial nucleus block the aversive motivational effect of both morphine and morphine withdrawal but spare morphine's discriminative effects. Behav.Neurosci. **110**:1496-1502.

443. Nader, K. and Van der Kooy, D. (1996) Clonidine antagonizes the aversive effects of opiate withdrawal and the rewarding effects of morphine only in opiate withdrawn rats. Behav.Neurosci. **110**:1-12.

444. Negus, S. S., Henriksen, S. J., Mattox, A., Pasternak, G. W., Portoghese, P. S., Takemori, A. E., Weinger, M. B., and Koob, G. F. (1993) Effect of antagonists selective fot mu, delta, and kappa opioid receptors on the reinforcing effects of heroin in rats. J.Pharmacol.exp.Ther. **265**:1245-1252.

445. Nemeth-Coslett, R. and Henningfield, J. E. (1986) Effects of nicotine chewing gum on cigarette smoking and subjective and physiologic effects. Clin. Pharmacol.Ther. **39**:625-630.

446. Nemeth-Coslett, R., Henningfield, J. E., O'Keeffe, M. K., and Griffiths, R. R. (1986) Effects of mecamylamine on human cigarette smoking and subjective ratings. Psychopharmacology **88**:420-425.

447. Nemeth-Coslett, R., Henningfield, J. E., O'Keeffe, M. K., and Griffiths, R. R. (1987) Nicotine gum: Dose-related effects on cigarette smoking and subjective ratings. Psychopharmacology **92**:424-430.

448. Newhouse, P. A., Sunderland, T., Narang, P. K., Mellow, A. M., Fertig, J. B., Lawlor, B. A., and Murphy, D. L. (1990) Neuroendocrine, physiologic, and behavioral responses following intravenous nicotine in nonsmoking healthy volunteers and in patients with Alzheimer's disease. Psychoendocrinol. **15**:471-484.

449. Nicolaides-Bouman, A., Wald, N., Forey, B., and Lee, P. (1993) International Smoking Statistics: A Collection of Historical Data from 22 Economically Developed Countries. Oxford University Press, London.

450. Nil, R. and Battig, K. (1989) Separate effects of cigarette smoke yield and smoke taste on smoking behaviour. Psychopharmacology **99**:54-59.

451. Nishida, N and Chiba, S. (1991) Intravenous self-administration of an enkephalin analog, EK-399, by rats. J.Toxicol.Sci. **16**:75-86.

452. NOP Omnibus Services. (1992) Smoking Habits 1991: A Report Prepared for the Department of Health. Department of Health, London.

453. Norman, R. (1975) Affective-cognitive consistency, attitudes, conformity, and behavior. J.Person.Soc.Psychol. **32**:83-91.

454. Nyberg, G., Panfilov, V., Sivertsson, R., and Wilhelmsen, L. (1982) Cardiovascular effect of nicotine chewing gum in healthy non-smokers. Eur.J.Clin.Pharmacol. **23**:303-307.

455. O'Brien, C. P. (1975) Experimental analysis of conditioning factors in human narcotic addiction. Pharmacol.Rev. **27**:533-543.

456. O'Brien, C. P., Childress, A. R., Ehrman, R., and Robbins, S. J. (1998) Conditioning factors in drug abuse: Can they explain compulsion? J.Psychopharmacol. **12**:15-22.

457. O'Neill, M. F., Dourish, C. T., and Iversen, S. D. (1991) Evidence for an involvement of D1 and D2 dopamine receptors in mediating nicotine-induced hyperactivity in rats. Psychopharmacology **104**:343-350.

458. Olds, J. (1956) Runway and maze behavior controlled by basomedial forebrain stimulation in the rat. J.Comp.Physiol.Psychol. **49**:507-512.

459. Olds, J. (1958) Satiation effects in self-stimulation of the brain. J.Comp.Physiol. Psychol. **51**:675-678.

460. Olds, J. and Milner, P. (1954) Positive reinforcement produced by electrical stimulation of septal area and other regions of the rat brain. J.Comp.Physiol. Psychol. **47**:419-427.

461. Olds, J. and Olds, M. E. (1965) Drives, reward, and the brain. In: Newcombe, T. M. (*Ed.*): New Directions in Psychology II. Holt, Rinehart, Winston, New York.

462. Olds, J. and Travis, R. P. (1960) Effects of chlorpromazine, meprobamate, pentobarbital, and morphine on self-stimulation. J.Pharmacol.exp.Ther. **128**:397-404.

463. Olds, M. E. (1976) Effectiveness of morphine and ineffectiveness of diazepam and phenobarbital on the motivational properties of hypothalamic self-stimulation behaviour. Neuropharmacol. **15**:117-131.

464. Olds, M. E. and Domino, E. F. (1969) Comparison of muscarinic and nicotinic cholinergic agonists on self-stimulation behavior. J.Pharmacol.exp.Ther. **166**:189-204.

465. Olds, M. E. and Domino, E. F. (1969) Differential effects of cholinergic agonists on self-stimulation and escape behavior. J.Pharmacol.exp.Ther. **170**:157-167.

466. Olive, K. E. and Ballard, J. A. (1996) Changes in employee smoking-behavior after implementation of restrictive smoking policies. Southern Med.J. **89**:699- 706.

467. Olmstead, M. C. and Franklin, K. B. (1994) Lesions of the pedunculopontine tegmental nucleus abolish catalepsy and locomotor depression induced by morphine. Brain Res. **662**:134-140.

468. Opitz, K. and Weischer, M. L. (1988) Volitional oral intake of nicotine in tupaias: Drug-induced alterations. Drug Alc.Depend. **21**:99-104.

469. Ossenkopp, K. P. and Guigno, L. (1990) Nicotine-induced conditioned taste aversions are enhanced in rats with lesions of the area postrema. Pharmacol. Biochem.Behav. **36**:625-630.

470. Owen, N. and Brown, S. L. (1991) Smokers unlikely to quit. J.Behav.Med. **14**:627-636.

471. Pagliusi, S. R., Tessari, M., DeVevey, S., Chiamulera, C., and Pich, E. M. (1996) The reinforcing properties of nicotine are associated with a specific patterning of c-fos expression in the rat brain. Eur.J.Neurosci. **8**:2247-2256.

472. Palmer, R. F. and Berens, A. (1983) Double-blind study of the effect of naloxone on the pleasure of smoking. Fed.Proc. **42**:654.

473. Parker, L. A. (1992) Place conditioning in a three-or-four choice apparatus: Role of stimulus novelty in drug-induced place conditioning. Behav.Neurosci. **106**:294-306.

474. Parker, L. A. and Gillies, T. (1995) THC-induced place and taste aversions in Lewis and Sprague-Dawley rats. Behav.Neurosci. **109**:71-78.

475. Parrott, A. C. and Craig, D. (1995) Psychological functions served by nicotine chewing gum. Addict.Behav. **20**:271-278.

476. Patkina, N. A. and Evartau, E. E. (1978) Rat behavior in an "open field" when chronically administered morphine. Farmakol.Toksikol. **41**:537-541.

477. Pavlov, I. P. (1927) Conditioned Reflexes. Oxford University Press, Oxford.

478. Peele, S. (1989) The Meaning of Addiction: Compulsive Experience and Its Interpretation . Lexington, Lexington.

479. Perkins, K. A., Amico, D. D., Sanders, M., Grobe, J. E., Wilson, A., and Stiller, R. L. (1996) Influence of training dose on nicotine discrimination in humans. Psychopharmacology 126:132-139.

480. Perkins, K. A., DiMarco, A., Grobe, J. E., Scierka, A., and Stiller, R. L. (1994) Nicotine discrimination in male and female smokers. Psychopharmacology 116: 407-413.

481. Perkins, K. A., Grobe, J. E., Epstein, L. H., Caggiula, A., Stiller, R. L., and Jacob, R. G. (1993) Chronic and acute tolerance to subjective effects of nicotine. Pharmacol.Biochem.Behav. 45:375-381.

482. Perkins, K. A., Grobe, J. E., Stiller, R. L., Fonte, C., and Goettler, J. E. (1992) Nasal spray nicotine replacement suppresses cigarette smoking desire and behavior. Clin.Pharmacol.Ther. 52:627-634.

483. Perkins, K. A., Grobe, J. E., Weiss, D., Fonte, C., and Caggiula, A. (1996) Nicotine preference in smokers as a function of smoking abstinence. Pharmacol. Biochem. Behav. 55:257-263.

484. Perkins, K. A., Sanders, M., Amico, D. D., and Wilson, A. (1997) Nicotine discrimination and self-administration in humans as a function of smoking status. Psychopharmacology 131:361-370.

485. Peterson, A. A., Campise, R. L., and Azrin, N. H. (1994) Behavioral and pharmacological treatments for tic and habit disorders: A review. J.Dev.Behav. Pediat. 15:430-440.

486. Petiti, D. B. and Friedman, G. D. (1983) Evidence for compensation in smokers of low yield cigarettes. Int.J.Epidemiology 12:487-489.

487. Petry, N. M. and Armentano, C. (1999) Prevalence, assessment, and treatment of pathological gambling: A review. Psychiat.Serv. 50:1021-1027.

488. Phillips, S. and Fox, P. (1998) An investigation into the effects of nicotine gum on short-term memory. Psychopharmacology 140:429-433.

489. Pich, E. M., Chiamulera, C., and Tessari, M. (1998) Neural substrate of nicotine addiction as defined by functional brain maps of gene expression. J.Physiol. (Paris) 92:225-228.

490. Pich, E. M., Pagliusi, S. R., Tessari, M., Talabot-Ayer, D., Hooft, van Huijsduijnen, and Chiamulera, C. (1997) Common neural substrates for the addictive properties of nicotine and cocaine. Science 275:83-86.

491. Pickworth, W. B., Bunker, E. B., and Henningfield, J. E. (1994) Transdermal nicotine: Reduction of smoking with minimal abuse liability. Psycho- pharmacology **115**:9-14.

492. Pickworth, W. B. and Fant, R. V. (1998) Endocrine effects of nicotine administration, tobacco and other drug withdrawal in humans. Psychoendocrinol. **23**:131-141.

493. Pickworth, W. B., Fant, R. V., Butschky, M. F., and Henningfield, J. E. (1997) Effects of mecamylamine on spontaneous EEG and performance in smokers and non-smokers. Pharmacol.Biochem.Behav. **56**:181-187.

494. Pidoplichko, V. I., DeBiasi, M., Williams, J. T., and Dani, J. A. (1997) Nicotine activates and desensitizes midbrain dopamine neurons. Nature **390**:401-404.

495. Pierce, J. P, Hatziandreu, E., and Flyer, P. (1989) Tobacco Use in 1986. Methods and Basic Tabulations from Adult Use of Tobacco Survey. Dept. of Health and Human Services, Centers for Disease Control, Office on Smoking and Health, Rockville, Maryland,

496. Pirke, K. M., Broocks, A., Wilckens, T., Marquard, R., and Schweiger, U. (1993) Starvation-induced hyperactivity in the rat: The role of endocrine and neurotransmitter changes. Neurosci.Biobehav.Rev. **17**:287-294.

497. Pliskoff, S. S. and Hawkins, T. D. (1963) Test of Deutsch's drive-decay theory of rewarding self-stimulation of the brain. Science **141**:823-824.

498. Pneu Michelin. (1995) Guide de Tourisme Jura.

499. Pneu Michelin. (1995) Guide de Tourisme Pays Rhenans "Rhin Superieur".

500. Pomerleau, C. S., Pomerleau, O. F., and Majchrzak, M. J. (1987) Mecamylamine pretreatment increases subsequent nicotine self-administration as indicated by changes in plasma nicotine level. Psychopharmacology **91**:391-393.

501. Pontieri, F. E., Tanda, G., Orzi, F., and DiChiara, G. (1996) Effects of nicotine on the nucleus accumbens and similarity to those of addictive drugs. Nature **382**:255-257.

502. Popper, K. R. (1963) Conjectures and Refutations. Routledge and Kegan Paul, London.

503. Powell, J. (1995) Conditioned responses to drug-related stimuli: Is context crucial? Addiction **90**:1089-1095.

504. Prada, J. A. and Goldberg, S. R. (1985) Effects of caffeine or nicotine pretreatments on nicotine self-administration by the squirrel monkey. Pharmacologist **27**:226.

505. Pradhan, S. N. (1970) Effects of nicotine on several schedules of behavior in rats. Arch.Int.Phamacodyn. **183**:127-138.

506. Pritchard, W. S., Robinson, J., Guy, T. D., Davis, R. A., and Stiles, M. F. (1996) Assessing the sensory role of nicotine in cigarette smoking. Psycho- pharmacology **127**:55-62.

507. Pritchard, W. S. and Robinson, J. H. (1996) Examining the relation between usual-brand nicotine yield, blood cotinine concentration and the nicotine "compensation" hypothesis. Psychopharmacology **124**:282-284.

508. Pullan, R. D., Rhodes, J., Ganesh, S., Mani, V., Morris, J. S., Williams, G. T., Newcombe, R. G., Russell, M. A. H., Feyerabend, C., Thomas, G. A. O., and Sawe, U. (1994) Transdermal nicotine for active ulcerative colitis. N.England J. Med. **330**:811-815.

509. Puustinen, P., Olkkonen, H., Kolonen, S., and Tuomisto, J. (1987) Microcomputer-aided measurement of puff parameters during smoking of low- and medium-tar cigarettes. Scand.J.Clin.Lab.Invest. **47**:655-660.

510. Quartermain, D. and Webster, D. (1968) Extinction following intracranial reward: The effect of delay between acquisition and extinction. Science **159**: 1259-1260.

511. Rachman, S. J. and Hodgson, R. (1980) Obsessions and Compulsions. Prentice-Hall, Englewood Cliffs, N.J.

512. Randall, C. K., Kraemer, P. J., and Bardo, M. T. (1998) Morphine-induced conditioned place preference in preweaning and adult rats. Pharmacol.Biochem. Behav. **60**:217-222.

513. Random House. (1980) The Random House College Dictionary, Revised Edition. Random House, New York.

514. Rasmussen, K., Czachura, J. F., Kallman, M. J., and Helton, D. R. (1996) The CCK-B antagonist LY288513 blocks the effects of nicotine withdrawal on the auditory startle. Neuroreport **7**:1050-1052.

515. Rasmussen, T. and Swedberg, M. D. (1998) Reinforcing effects of nicotinic compounds: Intravenous self-administration in drug-naive mice. Pharmacol. Biochem.Behav. **60**:567-573.

516. Rauhala, P., Idanpaan-Heikkila, J. J., Tuominen, R. K., and Mannisto, P. T. (1995) Differential disappearence of tolerance to thermal, hormonal and locomotor effects of morphine in the male rat. Eur.J.Pharmacol. **285**:69-77.

517. Ravizza, L., Maina, G., Bogetto, F., Albert, U., Barzega, G., and Bellino, S. (1998) Long term treatment of obsessive-compulsive disorder. CNS Drugs **10**:247-255.

518. Ray, O. (1978) Drugs, Society, and Human Behavior. C.V. Mosby Company, Saint Louis.

519. Reavill, C. and Stolerman, I. P. (1990) Locomotor activity in rats after administration of nicotinic agonists intracerebrally. Br.J.Pharmacol. **99**:273-278.

520. Reid, L. D., Hunsicker, J. P., Lindsay, J. L., Gallistel, C. R., and Kent, E. W. (1973) Incidence and magnitude of the 'priming effect' in self-stimulating rats. J.Comp.Physiol.Psychol. **82**:286-293.

521. Reid, M. S., Ho, I. B., and Berger, S. P. (1998) Behavioral and neurochemical components of nicotine sensitization following 15-day pretreatment: Studies on contextual conditioning. Behav.Pharmacol. **9**:137-148.

522. Revec, G. V., Grabner, C. P., Pierce, R. C., and Bardu, M. T. (1997) Transient increases in catecholaminergic activity in medial prefrontal cortex and nucleus accumbens shell during novelty. Neurosci. **76**:707-714.

523. Richmond, R. L. (1997) A comparison of measures used to assess effectiveness of the transdermal nicotine patch at 1 year. Addict.Behav. **22**:753-757.

524. Richmond, R. L., Harris, K., and de Almeida, N. A. (1994) The transdermal nicotine patch: Results of a randomized placebo-controlled trial. Med.J.Aust. **161**:130-135.

525. Riese, M. L. (1995) Mothers' ratings of infant tempermant: Relation to neonatal latency to soothe by pacifier. J.Genet.Psychol. **156**:23-31.

526. Risinger, F. O. and Oakes, R. A. (1995) Nicotine-induced conditioned place preference and conditioned place aversion in mice. Pharmacol.Biochem.Behav. **51**:457-461.

527. Risner, M. E. and Goldberg, S. R. (1983) A comparison of nicotine and cocaine self-administration in the dog: Fixed-ratio and progressive-ratio schedules of intravenous drug infusion. J.Pharmacol.exp.Ther. **224**:319-326.

528. Robbins, T. W., McAlonan, G., Muir, J. L., and Everitt, B. J. (1997) Cognitive enhancers in theory and practice: Studies of the cholinergic hypothesis of cognitive deficits in Alzheimer's disease. Behav.Brain Res. **83**:15-23.

529. Robinson, J., Pritchard, W. S., and Davis, R. A. (1992) Psychopharmacological effects of smoking a cigarette with typical "tar" and carbon monoxide yields but minimal nicotine. Psychopharmacology **108**:466-472.

530. Robinson, S. F., Marks, M. J., and Collins, A. C. (1996) Inbred mouse strains vary in oral self-selection of nicotine. Psychopharmacology **124**:332-339.

531. Ronis, D. L., Yates, J. F., and Kirscht, J. P. (1989) Attitudes, decisions, and habits as determinants of repeated behavior. In: Praktanis, A. R., Breckler, S. J., and Greenwald, A. G. (*Eds.*): Attitude Structure and Function. Lawrence Erlbaum Associates, Hilldale, N.J.

532. Rosa, M., Pacifici, R., Altieri, I., Pichini, S., Ottaviani, G., and Zuccaro, P. (1992) How the steady-state cotinine concentration in cigarette smokers is directly related to nicotine intake. Clin.Pharmacol.Ther. **52**:324-329.

533. Rose, J. E. (1984) Discriminablilty of nicotine in tobacco smoke: Implications for titration. Addict.Behav. **9**:189-193.

534. Rose, J. E. (1996) Nicotine addiction and treatment. Ann.Rev.Med. **47**:493-507.

535. Rose, J. E., Behm, F., and Levin, E. D. (1993) Role of nicotine dose and sensory cues in the regulation of smoke intake . Pharmacol.Biochem.Behav. **44**:891-900.

536. Rose, J. E., Behm, F. M., and Westman, E. C. (1998) Nicotine-mecamylamine treatment for smoking cessation: The role of precessation therapy. Exp.Clin. Psychopharmacol. **6**:331-343.

537. Rose, J. E., Behm, F. M., Westman, E. C., Levin, E. D., Stein, R. M., and Ripka, G. V. (1994) Mecamylamine combined with nicotine skin patch falicitates smoking cessation beyond nicotine patch treatment alone. Clin.Pharmacol.Ther. **56** :86-99.

538. Rose, J. E. and Corrigall, W. A. (1997) Nicotine self-administration in animals and humans: Similarities and differences. Psychopharmacology **130**:28-40.

539. Rose, J. E., Herskovic, J. E., Trilling, Y., and Jarvik, M. E. (1985) Transdermal nicotine reduces cigarette craving and nicotine preference. Clin.Pharmacol.Ther. **38**:450-456.

540. Rose, J. E. and Hickman, C. S. (1987) Citric acid aerosol as a potential smoking cessation aid. Chest **92**:1005-1008.

541. Rose, J. E. and Levin, E. D. (1991) Inter-relationships between conditioned and primary reinforcement in the maintenance of cigarette smoking. Br.J.Addict. **86**:605-609.

542. Rose, J. E., Sampson, A., Levin, E. D., and Henningfield, J. E. (1989) Mecamylamine increases nicotine preference and attenuates nicotine discrimination. Pharmacol.Biochem.Behav. **32**:933-938.

543. Rose, J. E., Zinser, M. C., Tashkin, D. P., Newcomb, R., and Ertle, A. (1984) Subjective response to cigarette smoking following airway anesthetization. Addict.Behav. **9**:211-215.

544. Rosecrans, J. A. (1969) Effects of nicotine on exploratory behaviour of female rats. Pharmacologist **11**:246.

545. Rosenberg, J., Benowitz, N. L., Jacob, P., and Wilson, K. M. (1980) Disposition kinetics and effects of intravenous nicotine. Clin.Pharmacol.Ther. **28**:517-522.

546. Rosenthal, R. J. and Lesieur, H. R. (1992) Self-reported withdrawal symptoms and pathological gambling. Am.J.Addict. **1**:150-154.

547. Routtenberg, A. (1968) "Self-starvation" of rats living in activity wheels: Adaptation effects. J.Comp.Physiol.Psychol. **66**:234-238.

548. Routtenberg, A. and Kuznesof, A. W. (1967) Self-starvation of rats living in activity wheels on a restricted feeding schedule. J.Comp.Physiol.Psychol. **64**: 414-421.

549. Rowlett, J. K., Wilcox, K. M., and Woolverton, W. L. (1998) Self-administration of cocaine-heroin combinations by rhesus monkeys: Antagonism by naltrexone. J.Pharmacol.exp.Ther. **286**:61-69.

550. Russell, M. A. H. (1976) Low-tar medium-nicotine cigarettes: A new approach to safer smoking. Br.Med.J.

551. Russell, M. A. H. (1989) Nicotine and the self-regulation of smoke intake. In: Wald, N. and Froggatt, P. (*Eds.*): Nicotine, Smoking and the Low Tar Programme. Oxford University Press, Oxford.

552. Russell, M. A. H., Jarvis, M., Iyer, M., and Feyerabend, C. (1980) Relation of nicotine yield of cigarettes to blood nicotine concentrations in smokers. Br.Med.J. **280**:972-976.

553. Russell, M. A. H., Jarvis, M. J., Feyerabend, C., and Saloojee, Y. (1986) Reduction of tar, nicotine, and carbon monoxide intake in low tar smokers. J.Epidemol.Commun.Hlth. **40**:80-85.

554. Russell, M. A. H., Sutton, S. R., Feyerabend, C., Cole, P. V., and Saloojee, Y. (1977) Nicotine chewing gum as a substitute for smoking. Br.Med.J. **23**:1060-1063.

555. Russell, M. A. H., Wilson, C., Patel, U. A., Cole, P. V., and Feyerabend, C. (1973) Comparison of the effect on tobacco consumption and carbon monoxide absorption of changing to high and low nicotine cigarettes. Br.Med.J. **4**:512-516.

556. Russell, M. A. H., Wilson, C., Patel, U. A., Cole, P. V., and Feyerabend, C. (1975) Plasma nicotine levels after smoking cigarettes with high, medium and low nicotine yields. Br.Med.J. **2**:414-416.

557. Rzewnicki, R. and Forgays, D. G. (1987) Recidivism and self-cure of smoking and obesity: An attempt to replicate. Am.Psychologist **42**:97-101.

558. Salamone, J. D., Cousins, M. S., and Snyder, B. J. (1997) Behavioral functions of nucleus accumbens dopamine: Empirical and conceptual problems with the anhedonia hypothesis. Neurosci.Biobehav.Rev. **21**:341-359.

559. Salin-Pascual, R., De, L. F., Gallicia-Polo, L., and Drucker-Colin, R. (1995) Effects of transdermal nicotine on mood and sleep in nonsmoking major depressed patients. Psychopharmacology **121**:476-479.

560. Sandborn, W. J., Tremaine, W. J., Offord, K. P., Lawson, G. M., Petersen, B. T., Batts, K. P., Croghan, I. T., Dale, L. C., Schroeder, D. R., and Hunt, R. D. (1997) Transdermal nicotine for mildly to moderately active ulcerative colitis. Ann.Intern.Med. **126**:364-371.

561. Sandwijk, J. P., Cohen, P. D. A., Musterd, S., and Langemeijer, M. P. S. (1995) Licit and Illicit Drug Use in Amsterdam II. Instituut voor Sociale Geografie Universiteit van Amsterdam, Amsterdam.

562. Sannerud, C. A., Prada, J., Goldberg, D. M., and Goldberg, S. R. (12-27-1994) The effects of sertraline on nicotine self-administration and food-maintained responding in squirrel monkeys. Eur.J.Pharmacol. **271**:461-469.

563. Santos, R. M. and Routtenberg, A. (1972) Attenuation of brain stimulation self-starvation: Adaptation effects. Physiol.Behav. **9**:831-837.

564. Satel, S. L. and Aeschbach, E. (1999) The Swiss Heroin Trials. J.Subst.Abuse **17**:331-335.

565. Saxena, K. and Scheman, A. (1985) Suicide plan by nicotine poisoining: A review of nicotine toxicity. Vet.Hum.Toxicol. **27**:495-497.

566. Schachter, S. (1982) Recidivism and self-cure of smoking and obesity. Am.Psychol. **37**:436-444.

567. Schaefer, G. J. and Holtzman, S. G. (8-16-1977) Dose- and time-dependent effects of narcotic analgesics on intracranial self-stimulation in the rat. Psychopharmacology **53**:227-234.

568. Schaefer, G. J. and Michael, R. P. (1981) Threshold differences for naloxone and naltrexone in the hypothalamus and midbrain using fixed ratio brain self-stimulation in rats. Psychopharmacology **74**:17-22.

569. Schaefer, G. J. and Michael, R. P. (1983) Morphine withdrawal produces differential effects on the rate of lever-pressing for brain self-stimulation in the hypothalamus and midbrain in rats. Pharmacol.Biochem.Behav. **18**:571-577.

570. Schaefer, G. J. and Michael, R. P. (1985) The discriminative stimulus properties and detection thresholds of intracranial self-stimulation: Effects of d-amphetamine, morphine, and haloperidol. Psychopharmacology **85**:289-294.

571. Schaefer, G. J. and Michael, R. P. (1986) Changes in response rates and reinforcement thresholds for intracranial self-stimulation during morphine withdrawal. Pharmacol.Biochem.Behav. **25**:1263-1269.

572. Schaefer, G. J. and Michael, R. P. (1986) Task-specific effects of nicotine in rats. Intracranial self-stimulation and locomotor activity. Neuropharmacol. **25**:125- 131.

573. Schaefer, G. J. and Michael, R. P. (1990) Interactions of naloxone with morphine, amphetamine and phencyclidine on fixed interval responding for intracranial self-stimulation in rats. Psychopharmacology **102**:263-268.

574. Schaefer, G. J. and Michael, R. P. (1992) Interactions between alcohol and nicotine on intracranial self-stimulation and locomotor activity in rats. Drug Alc. Depend. **30**:37-47.

575. Schechter, M. D. and Rosecrans, J. A. (1972) Nicotine as a discriminative cue in rats: Inability of related drugs to produce a nicotine-like effect. Psychopharmacologia **27**:379-387.

576. Schenk, S., Coupal, A., Williams, T., and Shizgal, P. (1981) A within-subject comparison of the effects of morphine on lateral hypothalamic and central gray self-stimulation. Pharmacol.Biochem.Behav. **15**:37-41.

577. Scherer, G. (1999) Smoking behaviour and compensation: A review of the literature. Psychopharmacology **145**:1-20.

578. Schilstrom, B., Svensson, H. M., Svensson, T. H., and Nomikos, G. G. (1998) Nicotine and food induced dopamine release in the nucleus accumbens of the rat: Putative role of alpha7 nicotinic receptors in the ventral tegmental area. Neurosci. **85**:1005-1009.

579. Schlatter, J. and Battig, K. (1979) Differential effects of nicotine and amphetamine on locomotor activity and maze exploration in two rat lines. Psychopharmacology **64**:155-161.

580. Schneider, N. G. and Jarvik, M. E. (1984) Time course of smoking withdrawal symptoms as a function of nicotine replacement. Psychopharmacology **82**:143-144.

581. Schneider, N. G., Lunell, E., Olmstead, R. E., and Fagerstrom, K. O. (1996) Clinical pharmacokinetics of nasal nicotine delivery. A review and comparison to other nicotine systems. Clin.Pharmacokinet. **31**:65-80.

582. Schneider, N. G., Olmstead, R., and Mody, F. (1995) Efficacy of a nasal nicotine spray in smoking cessation: A placebo-controlled, double-blind trial. Addiction **90**:1671-1682.

583. Schneider, W. and Shiffrin, R. M. (1977) Controlled and automatic human information processing: I. Detection, search, and attention. Psychol.Rev. **84**:1- 66.

584. Schulteis, G., Markou, A., Gold, L. H., Stinus, L., and Koob, G. F. (1994) Relative sensitivity to naloxone of multiple indices of opiate withdrawal: A quantitative dose-response analysis. J.Pharmacol.exp.Ther. **271**:1391-1398.

585. Schultz, W. (1997) Dopamine neurons and their role in reward mechanisms. Cur.Opin.Neurobiol. **7**:191-197.

586. Schultz, W., Dayan, P. R., and Montague, P. R. (1997) A neural substrate of prediction and reward. Science **275**:1593-1599.

587. Schwartz, J. L. (1987) Review and evaluation of smoking cessation methods: The United States and Canada, NIH Publication No.87-2940, Washington, DC, US Department of Health and Human Services.,

588. Schwid, S. R., Hirvonen, M. D., and Keesey, R. E. (1992) Nicotine effects on body weight: A regulatory perspective. Am.J.Clin.Nutr. **55**:878-884.

589. Segura-Torres, P., Portell-Cortes, I., and Morgado-Bernal, I. (1991) Improvement of shuttle-box avoidance with post-training intracranial self-stimulation in rats: A parametric study. Behav.Brain Res. **28**:161-167.

590. Sepkovic, D. W., Parker, K., Axelrad, C. M., Haley, N. J., and Wynder, E. L. (1984) Cigarette smoking as a risk of cardiovascular disease. Part V. Biochemical parameters with increased and decreased nicotine content cigarettes. Addict.Behav. **9**:255-263.

591. Serdula, M. K., Mokdad, A. H., Pamuk, E. R., Williamson, D. F., and Byers, T. (1995) Effects of question order on estimates of the prevalence of attempted weight loss. Am.J.Epidemiol. **142**:64-67.

592. Serdula, M. K., Williamson, D. F., Anda, R. F., Levy, A., Heaton, A., and Byers, T. (1994) Weight control practices in adults: Results of a multistate telephone survey. Am.J.Pub.Health **84**:1821-1824.

593. Seward, J. P., Uyeda, A. A., and Olds, J. (1959) Resistance to extinction following cranial self-stimulation. J.Comp.Physiol.Psychol. **52**:294-299.

594. Shaffer, H. J. (1997) The most important unresolved issue in the addictions: Conceptual chaos. Substance Use and Misuse **32**:1573-1580.

595. Shaham, Y., Adamson, L. K., Grocki, S., and Corrigall, W. A. (1997) Reinstatement and spontaneous recovery of nicotine seeking in rats [published erratum appears in Psychopharmacology 1997 Sep;133(1):106]. Psycho- pharmacology **130**:396- 403.

596. Sherman, J. E., Pickman, C., Rice, A., Liebeskind, J. C., and Holman, E. W. (1980) Rewarding and aversive effects of morphine: temporal and pharmacological properties. Pharmacol.Biochem.Behav. **13**:501-515.

597. Sherman, J. E., Roberts, T., Roskam, S. E., and Holman, E. W. (1980) Temporal properties of the rewarding and aversive effects of amphethamine in rats. Pharmacol.Biochem.Behav. **13**:597-599.

598. Shiffman, S. (1989) Tobacco "chippers": Individual differences in tobacco dependence. Psychopharmacology **97**:535-538.

599. Shiffman, S., Fischer, L. B., Zettler-Segal, M., and Benowitz, N. (1990) Nicotine exposure among nondependent smokers. Arch.Gen.Psychiatry **47**:333-336.

600. Shiffrin, R. M. and Schneider, W. (1977) Controlled and automatic human information processing: II. Perceptual learning, automatic attending, and a general theory. Psychol.Rev. **84**:127-190.

601. Shoaib, M., Schindler, C. W., and Goldberg, S. R. (1997) Nicotine self-administration in rats: Strain and nicotine pre-exposure effects on acquisition. Psychopharmacology **129**:35-43.

602. Shoaib, M. and Stolerman, I. P. (1996) Brain sites mediating the discriminative stimulus effects of nicotine in rats. Behav.Brain Res. **78**:183-188.

603. Shoaib, M. and Stolerman, I. P. (1999) Plasma nicotine and cotinine levels following intravenous nicotine self-administration in rats. Psychopharmacology **143**:318-321.

604. Shoaib, M., Stolerman, I. P., and Kumar, R. (1994) Nicotine-induced place preferences following prior nicotine exposure in rats. Psychopharmacology **113**: 445-452.

605. Shoaib, M., Swanner, L. S., Yasar, S., and Goldberg, S. R. (1999) Chronic caffeine exposure potentiates nicotine self-administration in rats. Psycho- pharmacology **142**:327-333.

606. Shuster, L. (1971) Tolerance and physical dependence. In: Clouet, D. H. (*Ed.*): Narcotic Drugs: Biochemical Pharmacology. Plenum Press, New York.

607. Siegel, M., Nelson, D. E., Peddicord, J. P., Merritt, R. K., Giovino, G. A., and Eriksen, M. P. (1996) The extent of cigarette brand and company switching: Results from the adult use-of-tabacco survey. Am.J.Preventive.Med. **12**:14-16.

608. Silagy, C., Mant, D., Fowler, G., and Lodge, M. (1994) Meta-analysis on efficacy of nicotine replacement therapies in smoking cessation. The Lancet **343**:139-142.

609. Singer, G., Simpson, F., and Lang, W. J. (1978) Schedule induced self-injection of nicotine with recovered body weight. Pharmacol.Biochem.Behav. **9**:387-389.

610. Singer, J. and Janz, T. (1990) Apnea and seizures caused by nicotine ingestion. Pediatr.Emerg.Care **6**:135-137.

611. Skinner, B. F. (1938) The Behavior of Organisms. Appleton-Century-Crofts, New York.

612. Slifer, B. L. and Balster, R. L. (1985) Intravenous self-administration of nicotine: With and without schedule-induction. Pharmacol.Biochem.Behav. **22**:61-69.

613. Smith, A. and Roberts, D. C. (1995) Oral self-administration of sweetened nicotine solutions by rats. Psychopharmacology **120**:341-346.

614. Smith, B. A., Fillion, T. J., and Blass, M. E. (1990) Orally mediated sources of calming in 1 to 3-day-old human infants. Dev.Psychol. **26**:731-737.

615. Smith, C. A. and Holman, E. W. (1987) Rewarding and aversive effects of stimulant drugs in infant rats. Pharmacol.Biochem.Behav. **26**:211-215.

616. Smith, L. A. and Lang, W. J. (1980) Changes occurring in self-administration of nicotine by rats over a 28-day period. Pharmacol.Biochem.Behav. **13**:215-220.

617. Smith, T. A., House, R. F., Croghan, I. T., Gauvin, T. R., Colligan, R. C., Offord, K. P., Gomez-Dahl, L. C., and Hurt, R. D. (1996) Nicotine patch therapy in adolescent smokers. Pediatrics **98**:659-667.

618. Solomon, R. (1977) The evolution of non medical opiate use in Canada. II.: 1930-1970. Drug Forum **6**:1-25.

619. Sonnedecker, G. (1956) Emergence and concept of the addiction problem. In: Livingston, R. B. (*Ed.*): Narcotic Drug Addiction Problems. Public Health Service, Bethesda, MD.

620. Sorg, B. A. and Kalivas, P. W. (1991) Effects of cocaine and footshock stress on extracellular dopamine levels in the ventral striatum. Brain Res. **559**:29-36.

621. Soria, R., Stapleton, J., Gilson, S. F., Sampson-Cone, A., Henningfield, J. E., and London, E. D. (1996) Subjective and cardiovascular effects of intravenous nicotine in smokers and non-smokers. Psychopharmacology **128**:221-226.

622. Spatz, C. and Jones, S. D. (1971) Starvation anorexia as an explanation of "self-starvation" of rats living in activity wheels. J.Comp.Physiol.Psychol. **77**:313-317.

623. Spealman, R. D. and Goldberg, S. R. (1982) Maintenance of schedule-controlled behavior by intravenous injections of nicotine in squirrel monkeys. J.Pharmacol. exp.Ther. **223**:402-408.

624. Spigelman, M. N., McLeod, W. S., and Rockman, G. E. (1991) Caloric vs. pharmacologic effects of ethanol consumption on activity anorexia in rats. Pharmacol.Biochem.Behav. **39**:85-90.

625. Spyraki, C., Fibiger, H. C., and Phillips, A. G. (1982) Dopaminergic substrates of amphetamine-induced place preference conditioning. Brain Res. **253**:185-193.

626. Srivastava, E. D., Russell, M. A. H., Feyerabend, C., Masterson, J. G., and Rhodes, J. (1991) Sensitivity and tolerance to nicotine in smokers and nonsmokers. Psychopharmacology **105**:63-68.

627. Stapleton, J. A., Russell, M. A. H., Feyerabend, C., Wiseman, S. M., Gustavsson, G., Sawe, U., and Wisemen, D. (1995) Dose effects and predictors of outcome in a randomized trial of transdermal nicotine patches in general practice. Addiction **90**:31-42.

628. Stein, L. (1958) Secondary reinforcement established without subcortical stimulation. Science **127**:466-467.

629. Stein, L. (1964) Reciprocal action of reward and punishment. In: Heath, R. G. (*Ed.*): The Role of Pleasure in Behavior. Hoeber, New York.

630. Stepney, R. (1981) Would a medium-nicotine, low-tar cigarette be less hazardous to health? Br.Med.J. **283**:1292-1296.

631. Stolerman, I. P. (1999) Inter-species consistency in the behavioural pharmaco- logy of nicotine dependence. Behav.Pharmacol. **10**:559-580.

632. Stolerman, I. P., Bunker, P., and Jarvik, M. E. (1974) Nicotine tolerance in rats: Role of dose and dose interval. Psychopharmacologia **34**:317-324.

633. Stolerman, I. P., Fink, R., and Jarvik, M. E. (1973) Acute and chronic tolerance to nicotine measured by activity in rats. Psychopharmacologia **30**:329-342.

634. Stolerman, I. P., Goldfarb, T., Fink, R., and Jarvik, M. E. (1973) Influencing cigarette smoking with nicotine antagonists. Psychopharmacologia **28**:247-259.

635. Stolerman, I. P. and Jarvis, M. J. (1995) The scientific case that nicotine is addictive. Psychopharmacology **117**:2-10.

636. Stolerman, I. P., Naylor, C., Elmer, G. I., and Goldberg, S. R. (1999) Discrimination and self-administration of nicotine by inbred strains of mice. Psychopharmacology **141**:297-306.

637. Strain, E. C., Bigelow, G. E., Liebson, I. A., and Stitzer, M. L. (1999) Moderate- vs high-dose methadone in the treatment of opioid dependence. JAMA **281**:1000-1005.

638. Stutz, R. M., Lewin, I., and Rocklin, R. W. (1965) Generality of drive decay as an explanatory concept. Psychonom.Sci. **2**:127-128.

639. Sugimoto, Y., Yamada, J., and Noma, T. (1998) Effects of anxiolitics, diazepam and tandospirone, on immobilization stress-induced hyperglycemia in mice. Life Sci. **63**:1221-1226.

640. Sutherland, G., Stapleton, J. A., Russell, M. A., and Feyerabend, C. (1995) Naltrexone, smoking behaviour and cigarette withdrawal. Psychopharmacology **120**:418-425.

641. Sutherland, G., Stapleton, J. A., and Russell, M. A. H. (1992) Randomised controlled trial of nasal nicotine spray in smoking cessation. Lancet **340**:324- 329.

642. Sutton, S. (1998) Predicting and explaining intentions and behavior: How well are we doing? J.Appl.Soc.Psychol. **28**:1317-1338.

643. Sutton, S., McVey, D., and Glanz, A. (1998) A comparative test of the theory of reasoned action and the theory of planned behavior in the prediction of condom use intentions in a national sample of English young people. Hlth.Psychol. **18**:72-81.

644. Sutton, S. R., Feyerabend, C., Cole, P. V., and Russell, M. A. H. (1978) Adjustment of smokers to dilution of tobacco smoke by ventilated cigarette holders. Clin.Pharmacol.Ther. **24**:395-405.

645. Sutton, S. R., Russell, M. A. H., Iyer, R., Feyerabend, C., and Saloojee, Y. (1982) Relationship between cigarette yields, puffing patterns, and smoke intake: Evidence for tar compensation? Br.Med.J. **28**:603.

646. Swedberg, M. D. B., Henningfield, J. E., and Goldberg, S. R. (1988) Evidence of nicotine dependency from animal studies: Self-administration. Tolerance and withdrawal. In: Russell,M.A.H., Stolerman, I.P., Wannacott, S.(Eds.) Nicotine: Actions and Medical Implications. Oxford, Oxford University Press. C.f. US Department of Health and Human Services, 1988.

647. Takayasu, T., Ohshima, T., Lin, Z., Nishigami, J., Nakaya, T., Maeda, H., and Tanaka, N. (1992) An autopsy case of fatal nicotine poisoning. Nippon Hoigaku Zasshi **46**:327-332.

648. Tang, J. L., Law, M., and Wald, N. (1994) How effective is nicotine replacement therapy in helping people to stop smoking? Br.Med.J. **308**:21-26.

649. Taylor, P. (1990) Agents acting at the neuromuscular junction and autonomic ganglis. In: Goodman Gilman, A., Rall, T. W., Nies, A. S., and Taylor, P. (*Eds.*): Goodman and Gilman's The Pharmacological Basis of Therapeutics. Pergamon Press, New York.

650. Ternes, J. W., O'Brien, C. P., Greenstein, R., and McLellan, A. T. (1980) Unreinforced self-injections: Effects of rituals and outcome in heroin addicts. In: Harris, L. S. (*Ed.*): Problems of Drug Dependence, 1979. US Government Printing Office, Washington DC.

651. Tessari, M., Valerio, E., Chiamulera, C., and Beardsley, P. M. (1995) Nicotine reinforcement in rats with histories of cocaine self-administration. Psychopharmacology **121**:282-283.

652. Thomas, G. A. O., Davies, S. V., Rhodes, J., Russell, M. A. H., Feyerabend, C., and Sawe, U. (1995) Is transdermal nicotine associated with cardiovascular risk? J.Royal Coll.Physicians of London **29**:392-396.

653. Thomas, G. A. O., Rhodes, J., Mani, V., Williams, G. T., Newcombe, R. G., Russell, M. A. H., and Feyerabend, C. (1995) Transdermal nicotine as maintenance therapy for ulcerative colitis. N.England J.Med. **13**:988-992.

654. Thompson, G. H. and Hunter, D. A. (1998) Nicotine replacement therapy. Ann.Pharmacother. **32**:1067-1075.

655. Tiffany, S. T. and Carter, B. (1998) Is craving the source of compulsive drug use? J.Psychopharmacol. **12**:23-30.

656. Tloczynski, J., Malinowski, A., and Lamorte, R. (1997) Rediscovering and reapplying contingent informal meditation. Int.J.Psychol.Orient **40**:14-21.

657. Tobacco Advisory Group of The Royal College of Physicians (2000) Nicotine Addiction in Britain. Royal College of Physicians, London.

658. Tobin, M. J. and Sackner, M. A. (1982) Monitoring smoking patterns of low and high tar cigarettes with inductive plethysmography. Am.Rev.Respir.Dis. **126**: 258-264.

659. Transdermal Nicotine Study Group (1991) Transdermal nicotine for smoking cessation. Six-months results from two multicenter controlled clinical trials. JAMA **266**:3133-3138.

660. Tsibul'skii, V. L. and Koval'zon, V. M. (1977) Effect of the "rapid" phase of sleep on self stimulation of the hypothalamus and septum in white rats. Zh.Vyssh.Deiat. **27**:792-800.

661. Turenne, S. D., Miles, C., Parker, L. A., and Siegel, S. (1996) Individual differences in reactivity to the rewarding/aversive properties of drugs: Assessment by taste and place conditioning. Pharmacol.Biochem.Behav. **53**: 511-516.

662. Turner, J. A. M., Sillett, R. W., and Ball, K. P. (1974) Some effects of changing to low-tar and low-nicotine cigarettes. Lancet **2**:737-739.

663. Urca, G. and Frenk, H. (1980) Pro- and anticonvulsant action of morphine in rats. Pharmacol.Biochem.Behav. **13**:343-347.

664. US Department of Health and Human Services (1964) Smoking and Health: report of the Advisory Committee to the Surgeon General of the public Health Services,

665. US Department of Health and Human Services. (1988) Nicotine Addiction: A Report of the Surgeon General, DHHS Publication Number (CDC) 88-8406. US Department of Health and Human Services, Office of the Assistant Secretary for Health, Rockville, MD: Office on Smoking and Health.

666. Valenstein, E. S. (1966) The anatomical locus of reinforcement. In: Stellar, E. and Sprague, J. M. (*Eds.*): Progress in Physiological Psychology. Academic Press, New York.

667. Valentine, J. D., Hokanson, J. S., Matta, S. G., and Sharp, B. M. (1997) Self-administration in rats allowed unlimited access to nicotine. Psychopharmacology **133**:300-304.

668. Van der Heyden, J. A., Zethof, T. J., and Olivier, B. (1997) Stress-induced hyperthermia in singly housed mice. Physiol.Behav. **62**:463-470.

669. Van der Kooy, D., Schiff, B. B., and Steele, D. (1978) Response-dependent effects of morphine on reinforcing lateral hypothalamic self-stimulation. Psychopharmacology **58**:63-67.

670. Van Dijk, A. P. M., Meijssen, M. A. C., Brouwer, A. J. B. W., Hop, W. C. J., van Bergeijk, J. D., Feyerabend, C., Wilson, J. H. P., and Zijlstra, F. J. (1998) Transdermal nicotine inhibits interleukin 2 synthesis by mononuclear cells derived from healthy volunteers. Eur.J.Clin.Investig. **28**:664-671.

671. Van Wolfswinkel, L. and Van Ree, J. M. (1985) Effects of morphine and naloxone on thresholds of ventral tegmental electrical self-stimulation. Naunyn Schmiedebergs Arch.Pharmacol. **330**:84-92.

672. Vanderschuren, L. J., Tjon, G. H., Nestby, P., Mulder, A. H., Schoffelmeer, A. N., and De Vries, T. J. (1997) Morphine-induced long-term sensitization to the locomotor effects of morphine and amphetamine depends on the temporal pattern of the pretreatment regimen. Psychopharmacology **131**:115-122.

673. Vasko, M. R. and Domino, E. F. (1978) Tolerance development to the biphasic effects of morphine on locomotor activity and brain acetylcholine in the rat. J.Pharmacol.exp.Ther. **207**:848-858.

674. Vela, G, Martin, S., Garcia-Gil, L., Crespo, J. A., Ruiz-Gayo, M., Fernandez- Ruiz, J. J., Garcia-Lecumberri, C., Pelaprat, D., Fuentes, J. A., Ramos, J. A., and Ambrosio, E. (1998) Maternal exposure to delta^9-tetrahydrocannabinol facilitates morphine self-administration behavior and changes regional binding to cetral mu opioid receptors in adult offspring female rats. Brain Res. **807**:101-109.

675. Villaneuva, H. F., Arezo, S., James, J. R., and Rosecrans, J. A. (1990) Withdrawal from chronic nicotine fails to produce a conditioned taste aversion to saccharin in rats. Pharmacol.Biochem.Behav. **37**:59-61.

676. Villaneuva, H. F., James, J. R., Arezo, S., and Rosecrans, J. A. (1991) Withdrawal from nicotine fails to produce a conditioned taste aversion to saccharine in rats and mice. NIDA Res.Monogr **105**:433-434.

677. Viswesvaran, C. and Schmidt, F. L. (1992) A meta-analytic comparison of the effectiveness of smoking cessation methods. J.Appl.Psychol. **77**:554-561.

678. Vives, F. and Mora, F. (1986) Effects of agonists and antagonists of cholinergic receptors on self-stimulation of the medial prefrontal cortex of the rat. Gen. Pharmacol. **17**:63-67.

679. Wakasa, Y., Takada, K., and Yanagita, T. (1995) Reinforcing effect as a function of infusion speed in intravenous self-administration of nicotine in rhesus monkeys. Nihon Shinkei Seishin Yakurigaku Zasshi **15**:53-59.

680. Wald, N. J., Idle, M., and Boreham, J. (1981) The importance of tar and nicotine in determining cigarette smoking habits. J.Epidemol.Commun.Hlth. **35**:23-24.

681. Warburton, D. M. (1985) Addiction, dependence and habitual substance use. Bulletin of the British Psychological Society **38**:285-288.

682. Warburton, D. M. (1989) Is nicotine use an addiction? Bulletin of the British Psychological Society **4**:166-170.

683. Warburton, D. M. (1989) Is nicotine use an addiction? The Psychologist: Bulletin of the British Psychological Society **4**:166-170.

684. Warburton, D. M. (1992) Nicotine as a cognitive enhancer. Prog. Neuropsycho-pharmacol.Biol. **16**:181-191.

685. Warburton, D. M. and Mancuso, G. (1998) Evaluation of the information processing and mood efffects of a transdermal nicotine patch. Psycho- pharmacology **135**:305-310.

686. Warburton, D. M. and Wesnes, K. (1984) Drugs as research tools in psychology: Cholinergic drugs and information processing. Neuropsychobiol. **11**:121-132.

687. Watanabe, K., Hara, C., and Ogawa, N. (1992) Feeding conditions and estrous cycle of female rats under the activity-stress preocedure from aspects of anorexia nervosa. Physiol.Behav. **51**:832.

688. Watkins, L. R., Wiertelak, E. P., McGorry, M., Martinez, J., Schwartz, B., Sisk, D., and Maier, S. F. (1998) Neurocircuitry of conditioned inhibition of analgesia: Effects of amygdala, dorsal raphe, ventral medullary, and spinal cord lesions on antianalgesia in the rat. Behav.Neurosci. **112**:360-378.

689. Watkins, S. S., Epping-Jordan, M. P., Koob, G. F., and Markou, A. (1999) Blockade of nicotine self-administration with nicotinic antagonists in rats. Pharmacol.Biochem.Behav. **62**:743-751.

690. Wauquier, A. and Niemegeers, C. J. (1976) Intracranial self-stimulation in rats as a function of various stimulus parameters. VI. Influence of fentanyl, piritramide, and morphine on medial forebrain bundle stimulation with monopolar electrodes. Psychopharmacologia **46**:179-183.

691. Wauquier, A., Niemegeers, C. J., and Lal, H. (1974) Differential antagonism by naloxone of inhibitory effects of haloperidol and morphine on brain self-stimulation. Psychopharmacologia **37**:303-310.

692. Weeks, J. R. and Collins, R. J. (1964) Factors affecting voluntary morphine intake in self-maintained addicted rats. Psychopharmacologia **6**:267-279.

693. Weibel, S. L. and Wolf, H. H. (1979) Opiate modification of intracranial self-stimulation in the rat. Pharmacol.Biochem.Behav. **10**:71-78.

694. Weihrauch, T. R. and Gauler, T. C. (1999) Placebo-efficacy and adverse effects in controlled clinical trials. Arzneimittelforschung **49**:385-393.

695. Weltzl, H., Alessandri, B., Oettinger, R., and Battig, K. (1988) The effects of long-term nicotine treatment on locomotion, exploration and memory in young and old rats. Psychopharmacology **96**:317-323.

696. Wen, H. L. and Ho, W. K. (1982) Suppression of withdrawal symptomps by dynorphin in heroin addicts. Eur.J.Pharmacol. **82**:183-186.

697. Wenzel, J. and Kuschinsky, K. (1990) Effects of morphine on gamma- aminobutyric acid turnover in the basal ganglia. Possible correlation with its biphasic action on motility. Arzneimittelforschung **40**:811-813.

698. Wesnes, K., Pitkethly, G. M., and Warburton, D. M. (1978) Oral nicotine preload and smoking behavior. C.f. Warburton, D.M. (1985) Nicotine and the smoker. Rev.Environ.Health **5**:343-390.

699. West, R. J., Russell, M. A. H., Jarvis, M. J., and Feyerabend, C. (1984) Does switching to an ultra-low nicotine cigarette induce nicotine withdrawal effects? Psychopharmacology **84**:120-123.

700. Wester, W. C. (1991) Habits. In: O'Grady, D. J. et al. (*Eds.*): Clinical Hypnosis with Children. New York.

701. Westman, E. C., Behm, F. M., and Rose, J. E. (1995) Airway sensory replacement combined with nicotine replacement for smoking cessation. Chest **107**:1358-1364.

702. Wetzel, M. C. (1963) Self-stimulation aftereffects and runway performance in the rat . J.Comp.Physiol.Psychol. **56**:673-678.

703. Wewers, M. E., Dhatt, R., and Tejwani, G. A. (1998) Naltrexone administration affects ad libitum smoking behavior. Psychopharmacology **140**:185-190.

704. White, A. R., Resch, K. L., and Ernst, E. (1999) A meta-analysis of acupuncture techniques for smoking cessation. Tobacco Control **8**:393-397.

705. White, J. M. and Ganguzza, C. C. (1985) Effects of nicotine on schedule- controlled behavior. Role of fixed-interval length and modification by mecamylamine and chlorpromazine. Neuropharmacol. **24**:75-82.

706. White, N. (1996) Addictive drugs as reinforcers: Multiple partial actions on memory systems. Addiction **91**:921-949.

707. White, N. M. (1989) Reward or reinforcement: What's the difference? Neurosci. Biobehav.Rev. **13**:181-186.

708. Whitewood, G. (1997) Hypnotic intervention in the breaking of a thumb sucking habit. Austral.J.Clin.Hypnother. **18**:1-4.

709. Whitey, C. H., Papacosta, A. O., Swan, A. V., Fitzsimons, B. A., Ellard, G. A., Burney, P. G. J., Colley, J. R. T., and Holland, W. W. (1992) Respiratory effects of lowering tar and nicotine levels of cigarettes smoked by young male middle tar smokers. II. Results of a randomised controlled trial. J.Epidemol. Commun.Hlth. **46**:281-285.

710. WHO Expert Committee on Drug Dependence (1956) Seventh Report of the WHO Expert Committee on Addiction, No. 116.

711. WHO Expert Committee on Drug Dependence (1993) WHO Technical Report Series, No. 836.

712. Wiederholt, I. C. (1993) The psychodynamics of sex offenses and implications for treatment. J.Offender Rehab. **18**:19-24.

713. Wikler, A. (1976) Aspects of tolerance to and dependence on cannabis. Ann.N.Y. Acad.Sci. **282**:126-147.

714. Williams, D. I. and Lowe, G. (1972) Light reinforcement in the rat: The effects of continuous and discontinuous periods of apparatus familiarization. Quart.J.Exp.Psych. **24**:98-101.

715. Wilson, A. L., Langley, L. K., Monley, J., Bauer, T., Rottunda, S., McFalls, E., Kovera, C., and McCarten, J. R. (1995) Nicotine patches in Alzheimer's disease:

Pilot study on learning, memory, and safety. Pharmacol.Biochem.Behav. **51**:509-514.

716. Wilson, M. C., Hitomi, M., and Schuster, C. R. (1971) Psychomotor stimulant self administration as a function of dosage per injection in the rhesus monkey. Psychopharmacologia **22**:271-281.

717. Winders, S. E., Dykstra, T., Coday, M. C., Amos, J. C., Wilson, M. R., and Wilkins, D. R. (1992) Use of phenylpropanoline to reduce nicotine cessation weight gain in rats. Psychopharmacology **108**:501-506.

718. Wise, R. A. (1982) Neuroleptics and operant behavior: The anhedonia hypothesis. Behav.Brain Sci. **5**:39-87.

719. Wise, R. A. (1996) Addictive drugs and brain stimulation reward. Ann.Rev. Neurosci. **19**:319-340.

720. Wise, R. A. and Bozarth, M. A. (1987) A psychomotor stimulant theory of addiction. Psychol.Rev. **94**:469-492.

721. Wise, R. A., Leone, P., Rivest, R., and Leeb, K. (1995) Elevations of nucleus accumbens dopamine and DOPAC levels during intravenous heroin self-administration. Synapse **21**:140-148.

722. Wise, R. A., Spindler, J., De Wit, H., and Gerberg, G. J. (1978) Neuroleptic-induced 'anhedonia' in rats: Pimozide blocks reward quality of food. Science **201**:262-264.

723. Woodman, G., Newman, S. P., Pavia, D., and Clarke, S. W. (1987) The separate effects of tar and nicotine on the cigarette smoking manoeuvre. Eur.J.Respir.Dis. **70**:316-321.

724. Woodruff, T. J., Rosbrook, B., Pierce, J., and Glantz, S. A. (1993) Lower levels of cigarette consumption found in smoke-free workplaces in California. Archives of Internal Medicine **153**:1485-1493.

725. Woods, D. J. and Routtenberg, A. (1971) "Self-starvation" in activity wheels: Developmental and chlorpromazine interactions. J.Comp.Physiol.Psychol. **76**:84-93.

726. Woodward, M. and Tunstall-Pedoe, H. (1993) Self-titration of nicotine: Evidence from the Scottish Heart Health Study. Addiction **88**:821-830.

727. Woolf, A., Burkhart, K., Caraccio, T., and Litovitz, T. (1996) Self-poisoning among adults using multiple transdermal nicotine patches. J.Toxicol.Clin. Toxicol. **34**:691-698.

728. Woolf, A., Burkhart, K., Caraccio, T., and Litovitz, T. (1997) Childhood poisoning involving transdermal nicotine patches. Pediatrics **99**:E4.

729. Yanagita, T. (1977) Brief review on the use of self-administration techniques for predicting drug dependence potential. In: Thompson, T. and Unna, K. R. (*Eds.*):

Predicting Dependence Liability of Stimulant and Depressant Drugs. Baltimore University Park Press, Baltimore.

730. Yang, C., Wu, W. H., and Zbuzek, V. K. (1992) Antinociceptive effects of chronic nicotine and nociceptive effect of its withdrawal measured by hot-plate and tail-flick in rats. Psychopharmacology **106**:417-420.

731. Yaryura-Tobias, J. A. and Neziroglu, F. A. (1997) Behavioral Treatment of Obsessive-Compulsive Spectrum Disorders. Norton, New York.

732. Yeomans, J. and Baptista, M. (1997) Both nicotinic and muscarinic receptors in ventral tegmental area contribute to brain-stimulation reward. Pharmacol. Biochem. Behav. **57**:915-921.

733. Zacny, J. P. and Stitzer, M. L. (1988) Cigarette brand-switching: Effects on smoke exposure and smoking behavior. J.Pharmacol.exp.Ther. **246**:619-627.

734. Zarrindats, M. R. and Oveisi, M. R. (1997) Effects of monoamine receptor antagonists on nicotine-induced hypophagia in the rat. Eur.J.Pharmacol. **321**: 157-162.

Index

Date Due

APR 2 1 2004			
APR 5 2004			
APR 1 9 2006			
APR 1 0 2006			